BONDASSAGE

KINKY EROTIC MASSAGE TIPS FOR LOVERS

Jaeleen Bennis
& Eve Minax

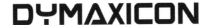

DYMAXICON

ISBN # 978-1-937965-19-8
Published by Dymaxicon
Sausalito, CA

www.dymaxicon.com

BONDASSAGE

Contents

WHAT IS BONDASSAGE?

*"Learning the art of Bondassage has opened up
a whole new aspect of my sensual side, teaching
me the importance of the connections we
can make without using words"—Jenna*

Imagine the last time you made love. Was it intense and exciting? Does it make you tingle thinking about it? More than likely it was routine, maybe kind of decent, or even downright awkward. Perhaps it has been so long you cannot remember? Your sexual practices do not have to be this way. If you are one of the lucky ones, then you are already having beautifully profound encounters, and you want more. There is always room to augment the hot sex you already have. If single, you can also more readily find new lovers who will share your interest in deeply connected sex.

Research shows that sexual intimacy does not occur in a vacuum; one must practice. When you are open and skillful in your intimate practices, you subliminally attract more lovers. By teaching you practical skills based on honest communication, sensual massage, basic bondage and kink, Bondassage® can help you expand your sexual repertoire, and consequently, (at the risk of sounding hyperbolic), change your life.

Bondassage combines innovative massage techniques with subtle breath and energy work, rhythmic body percussion, slow luxurious flogging, and a delicious menu of skilled sensation play. Created in 2008 by Certified Massage Therapist Jaeleen Bennis, the Bondassage program has enriched the professional practices of masseuses, bodyworkers and sex educators by offering training and certification in this unique set of practices. However, you don't need to be a professional practitioner to appreciate the benefits. You can read this book, follow the instructions, and learn to improve your erotic connections immensely.

We'll begin by giving you a basic grounding in simple massage techniques—the difference between our version and others out there being that our basics don't shy away from intimate contact. Next, we'll map the sensory landscape you will be exploring, emphasizing how the use of mild restraint and sensory deprivation, both hallmarks of the Bondassage experience, can serve to heighten the senses and increase pleasure. After that, once you're primed and ready, we'll introduce you to tools and techniques borrowed from the BDSM world that can send you and your partner rocketing to new heights of erotic stimulation. Lastly, after we've provided you with the toolkit and the skills, we give you some simple "recipes" to follow for building the perfect session for you and your partner, whatever your level of experience or sense of adventure.

Now, imagine yourself after learning the skills in this book: You meet your lover, restrain them lightly (or they you), and together you embark on a luscious journey of sensuality and orgasmic bliss. You take them to the edge and back again, over and again until they experience a crescendo of explosive pleasure, cathartic delights, deepening your connection and your love.

You have now entered the realm of Bondassage.

Let us explain further...

LETTING GO... THE ULTIMATE POWER

Ever wondered what it might be like to explore your sensual desires, to sexually surrender, to fully let go and give your power over to another? Perhaps you have fantasized about how it would be to take the erotic power given to you by another? Whether you're a novice or an experienced sexual explorer, combining light bondage, sensory deprivation, massage and sensation play will not only bring you excitement and pleasure, it will also deepen trust and love in your relationship. We are delighted to be your guides on this journey of submission, exploration and pleasure, and we anticipate some life-changing experiences for you.

Sexual surrender is the ultimate power, and the incredibly sensual art of Bondassage is unlike anything you've ever experienced or even imagined. To describe the awakenings it may stir, let's take a closer look at the picture. If you are the receiver, it all starts with you removing your clothes, finding yourself naked and kneeling, a leather collar around your neck and padded cuffs locked onto your wrists and ankles. You gaze longingly into your partner's eyes, they look at you with full acknowledgement of the power being exchanged, before your eyes are covered with a soft blindfold. Your partner, the giver, takes you, the receiver, gently over to a comfortable padded massage table (or bed), places headphones on your ears and allows you to sink deeply into your body as a selection of specially chosen erotic music plays through your headphones. You are then lightly secured, and your sensual erotic journey deepens...

As you surrender to the sensations and forget the outside world, you get taken to a place of exquisite enjoyment, a place where you can indulge your senses and embrace pleasure. Imagine warm hands working their way over your body... gently kneading, touching and stroking you all over. You find yourself deeply relaxing, and the depth of the relaxation permeates every part of your being. As you shed the stress and tension of the day, you drift into a new level of ecstasy. You're safe, you're happy, you're in complete bliss. You emerge relaxed and energized, more deeply connected with your partner, ready to take on the world!

Are you ready to discover a world of blissful intensity and intimacy?

"Masterful massage, sensual flogging,
fur mitts, feathers and light, wicked
spanking—I was in heaven."—Beth

SETTING THE SCENE: CREATING THE "BUBBLE"

"Bondassage sets forth structure. In the past, I had trouble planning—I was trying to do too much!"—Rachel

Due to stigmatism BDSM (Bondage & Discipline, Dominance & Submission, Sadism & Masochism) has been practiced secretly for eons, yet psychologists know that it is often through exploring and embracing the shadow side of ourselves that we find transformation and healing. A recent study from the Netherlands in the *Journal of Sexual Medicine* found that "the subjective well-being of BDSM participants was higher than that of the control group. Together, these findings suggest that BDSM practitioners are characterized by greater psychological and interpersonal strength and autonomy." Giving ourselves permission to explore these "dark" aspects of our sexual nature, especially in the context of a loving and consensual encounter, is one way of deepening our connection not only with a partner, but also with ourselves. By bringing the tools and techniques of BDSM play out of the dungeon and into the warm, candle-lit "bubble" of the massage room, (or bedroom), Bondassage makes this kind of play safe and accessible for anyone with a healthy curiosity about love, sexual energy and self-awareness.

With Bondassage, the atmosphere you create means just as much as the implements and techniques you utilize. Intention is everything in the art of sensual bodywork, so you want to insure the surroundings exemplify that intention. Ideally, your intention is to cultivate a mutual feeling of warmth and intimacy between you and your partner. BDSM practitioners commonly speak of an encounter as a "scene," terminology we think captures the carefully-crafted nature of a Bondassage encounter.

Intimacy and connection are easier to attain when the atmosphere is warm, dimly lit, and inviting, (music, colors, smells), to your partner. By setting the scene "just so," you create a bubble for the two of you (or more if you like!), to inhabit for the amount of time that you are together. The bubble offers a safe, sexy, open-hearted place for you to explore your wildest dreams. It's also a terrific place to enjoy yourselves without having to worry about looking for toys, or an extra towel, or even about your performance. Half of poor performance comes from being ill-prepared. Prepare yourself, prepare the space, and relax into each other; everyone will feel safer, more prioritized, and ready for action!

THE BASICS

Temperature

Most people feel most comfortable in a room that is at least 75 degrees warm while naked. Be sure to blast the furnace, stoke the fireplace, or turn the space heater on to insure the setting is warm and cozy.

Supplies

In order to get started with your Bondassage session, you will need some simple supplies; probably easily found in your home already, plus a couple extra items that you may need to procure in order to create a sensual, hands-on, care free, relaxing adventure for both of you.

Sheets

You may wish to designate a particular sheet for your playtime. Satin sheets are delicious, or try flannel or fleece sheets for variety.

Towels

You'll want two or three warm wet towels on hand for cleanup. These are easily created by placing a wet towel in a plastic bag and microwaving it for two or three minutes, then placing it in a thermal bag so that the towels maintain their soothing heat. Of course you can always create a warm, wet towel from the tap also!

Extra Dry Towels

For wiping down your receiver and general clean up.

Warm Massage Oil/Cream/Lotion

*Many sensual massage therapists swear by organic coco-
nut oil because of its wonderful smell and antibacterial/
anti-fungal properties. You can easily warm your massage
cream/oil by placing it in a container of hot water, or in
a crockpot with a bit of water at the bottom. In a pinch,
Jaeleen likes putting her massage cream (both of us love
Biotone Dual Purpose Massage Creme and Biotone Clear
Results Oil) in a glass container and popping it in the microwave for 20-25 seconds (uncovered).*

Bondage Gear and Toys

*We'll go into these important aspects of Bondassage in
greater detail later in this book, once you have more context for understanding their role. For now, it is enough to
know that the key is to begin your session prepared: Cut
relevant ropes and have them ready for use in session. If
using restraints, have them laid out or already locked onto
your bed or massage table. If you choose to incorporate
sensation play in your session, using items like feathers,
fur, floggers or sex toys., one rule of thumb is to always
test new or unfamiliar toys on yourself before using them
with your sexual partner. That could mean trying on the
blindfold or cuffs, taking a slapper on your forearm to feel
its intensity or perhaps using that special insertable toy to
see how penetrative it feels.*

Prep music

Choose music that doesn't distract and promotes relaxation. Many people prefer instrumental (non-vocal) music. We use ambient, slow-beat (60 bpm), music with non-English lyrics in our sessions. Wireless headphones are a joy to use—be sure to check the volume on the headphones your partner will be wearing. If using corded headphones, check to see that the cord will be out of the way.

Candles

Wax or LED candles and/or a dimmer switch on your light source evokes an erotic atmosphere. You might light some incense (as long as neither you nor your partner have a chemical/smell sensitivity).

Check your nails!

If they're even a bit scraggly, trim and file them (make sure to get the skin around the nails as well).

Now breathe, center yourself and smile!

ADDITIONAL SUPPLIES

A well-stocked nightstand contributes a lot toward helping your erotic play proceed smoothly. Rummaging through drawers, tramping off to the bathroom, or needing to make a quick trip to the kitchen can "pop the bubble" the two of you are creating. A small amount of planning ahead is well worth it. Assuming most of your sexual activity takes place in your bed, it would be helpful to keep these supplies nearby, perhaps in your nightstand or in a flat box underneath your bed. Eve keeps hers in a wide but not very deep container under the bed, fully stocked and ready to go at a moment's notice. Here are some suggestions for your "trousseau":

Personal Lubricant

Lube makes life easier (make sure to buy a lubricant with an easy-to-use bottle cap!). If you use water-soluble lubricants, also keep a small "finger bowl" of water handy so you can add a few drops as necessary. Don't add too much water, as doing so can flush most of the lubricant away from where it needs to be. Our preference is for silicone lube. More on that later.

Safer sex barriers

Gloves, finger cots, and condoms. Be aware if your partner has latex allergies and have a non-latex solution handy. Place 2 or 3 condoms or gloves over a vibrator or dildo, then simply remove one barrier at a time in order to move the toy from anus to vagina.

Tissues, wet wipes, hand sanitizer

For quick and easy clean ups that don't require more muscle.

Safety scissors

These have blunt tips to quickly cut ropes in an emergency, and are easily found at your local pharmacy or online.

Water
With bendable straws or in a drinking bottle, to share with your lover.

Chocolate / fresh fruit / finger foods
To revitalize and refresh. Also used as sensual play.

Cough drops, mints, or fresh mint
To help soothe the throat and keep breath fresh.

Blanket
For aftercare, the cool-down portion after your interlude.

Pillows
To place under your partner's hips and head.

Flashlight
In case of a power outage, you don't want to be fumbling to undo restraints in the dark. Don't forget the extra batteries and keep them updated.

Tupperware or a couple of gallon plastic bags
Any toy that needs cleaning goes into the bag so you can carry it without dirtying the other toys, many which can go straight to the dishwasher after a hot rinse first. Eve uses chux/disposable underpads or puppy pads and towels to keep used toys in a contained area during play.

Curiosity and a sense of humor
These will, of course, take you very far in your sexual journey.

PRE-PLAY DISCUSSION

Before bringing Bondassage elements into your play-time with a lover or potential sex partner, it's important that you both communicate your sexual wants and needs beforehand in order to ensure the psychological and physical safety of all parties involved. Unless you are highly experienced, or have played together often, negotiations ideally start *before* you even reach the bedroom. Even if you and your partner have played many times before, knowing how your partner is doing at that moment in their life can save embarrassing and unwanted outcomes. Remember also to keep your judgments in check and your compassion (for each of you) on hand. Some Suggestions:

> *Ask whether your partner has any previous BDSM/kink experience and if so, have them specify what they did and what worked and did not work for them. Keep it in mind that different people at different times have different boundaries, so you should have some flexibility here. Do respect all* **hard** *limits, things that your partner knows that they cannot tolerate. And remember, this is an exploration for both of you, so if you wish to merely start out with the sensual massage and a blindfold, then that is where you're at. Pushing to "do it all" will never make for better sensual exploration.*

> *Ask about any relevant medical issues (high blood pressure, blood sugar issues, prescription medications such as blood thinners, etc.). Sometimes men like taking vasodilators, (like Viagra), for erotic journeys. Ask! It's better to know than not.*

Make sure you know about any current injuries and illness (i.e. a rotator cuff injury would contraindicate tying the hands above the head, for instance) or old injuries. Knee replacements, hemorrhoids and even dental work could all be relevant. As far as STIs and STDs, you may have discussed that with your partner already with regard to sex, but if you are playing with toys, you will mostly be concerned with proper clean up. Covered toys are fairly safe from most STI's and STD's, especially when cleaned properly. We'll discuss toy clean up more in depth in a later chapter.

Ask about any allergies—especially latex and nuts, used in both safer sex barriers and massage oil made from co-conut oil, for example.

Ask if they are comfortable with internal (anal/vaginal) massage. If uncertain, offer to massage the outside gently and if they want more they can indicate to you accordingly. If not, please respect that as a hard limit (for now perhaps). Establish boundaries and together come up with a safe word ("mercy" is a nice classic). You may also consider green for "go!" yellow for "slow down," and red for "stop!" If you know each other well, you will still want to check in. How was your day? How are you feeling? Did anything happen today that might change your experience? (starting your period, looked over for a promotion, etc).

The above may sound like a lot of material to cover, and at first it may seem daunting. If you approach it as a shared conversation, however, you may be delighted to get those questions out of the way, get to know your partner more intimately, and actually get a little turned on by all the possibilities that remain!

To give you more information about how to keep your play safe and sexy, we want to insure you know some basic safety techniques. Visit bondassage.com for expanded safety information.

Should a situation arise during your play time, give your partner a brief apology, if that seems appropriate, then do what you can to move on to something else. There is probably little to be gained by stopping to argue or debate the point in depth, particularly right then. Save discussions for later.

On the other hand, if you are the receiver, and your partner starts to do something that really doesn't work for you, please diplomatically let them know that as soon as you can. Being "polite" in this situation may only allow your displeasure to build to uncontrollable levels. Speak up as soon as possible in a gentle but honest tone, saying something like "I'd prefer you not do that" or if an adjustment, "a little slower please." Remember, this is almost undoubtedly not willful misconduct on their part. They are probably doing it in an attempt, however misguided, to arouse you. Speak up, but give them the benefit of the doubt, especially if your partner is learning. As the giver, should your receiver speak up, it is best to say "thanks for telling me" or something along those lines and change it up. Even if it feels "forced" in the moment, everyone will feel more at ease later if no unnecessary hiccoughs occur.

"Bondassage is a leap of Faith. Zero to infinity in 60 minutes. It's way beyond stimulating and sensual, it's downright mind blowing."—Allen

SENSUAL MASSAGE 101

"I take pleasure in touching my lover and taking him to the edge. Each touch and sensation helps him experience relaxation and extreme exhilaration. I love how deeply he can surrender."—Lorna

THE BASICS

Note: Your partner may be someone with a penis or someone with a vulva... regardless of their gender. For ease of expression, the pronouns and adjectives used are "he" and "his" in the Penis Pleasure chapter, and "she" and "her" in the Boobie Bliss and Pussy Pleasuring chapters. In other parts of this book you'll see a combination of pronouns used, including the grammatically controversial "they" when gender is neutral. Our intention is to honor and include all genders, all genitalia and all anatomical descriptions while keeping the linguistic acrobatics to a graceful minimum.

Jaeleen has found it easier to learn new techniques by watching videos, and highly suggests that you take a look at Jaiya's Red Hot

Touch *videos on Amazon.com.*

Sensual massage is all about being present in the moment, with both your awareness and your touch. It's about how deeply and consciously you can go into the art of giving your partner pleasure. The art of receiving is about simply breathing and staying aware of what you are feeling in each moment. It is not a passive doormat position, rather a place of reception to your lover's energy.

Slowness itself is an incredible art, and we've lost the habit of it. When we move in slow, regular and harmonious movements, awareness finds its place. Attention is heightened. Your body begins to enjoy the tiniest things.

Put away all the clutter of your everyday life. Set a romantic atmosphere with candles and relaxing music. Make sure the room is warm enough so that your partner won't be cold. Have everything that you might need nearby—extra towels, warmed oil (try placing a small container of it in a cup of hot water).

If at all possible, purchase a massage table with adjustable legs. Jaeleen likes to have her table on the lowest setting so it's easy for her to climb up on. If cost is a factor, you can always find used massage tables in the classifieds or on the Internet. A massage table is one of the best investments you can make, and it easily converts to a bondage table by simply installing eye bolts down the sides.

If a massage table isn't handy, you can use a firm surface like a floor that you've covered with a few blankets. Jaeleen likes to put a couple of large pillows (or a full-body pillow) under the chest, belly and hips. Eve uses a fold out futon that stores easily. Being lower is a comfortable position for the receiver, gives you better access to their body, and reduces strain on their neck.

Sensual massage is all about tease and denial, and the power of slow, soft, deliberate touch to relax and build arousal. Take your cues from your lover's breathing and their reactions. Touch for your own pleasure, and do only what pleases you. Use different pressures and degrees of slowness, and change them periodically. Alternate high-energy strokes with more mellow ones. Mix it up, keep your partner guessing!

The secret to an incredibly sensuous massage is touching with your whole hand. Touch that is centered in the fingertips can feel more like poking than a caress. To fix this, as the giver, simply shift your focus from your fingertips to the palm of your hand. Find the small indentation in the middle of your palm: that's the "heart" of your palm. Place the heart of the palm first, then let the rest of your hand relax. When you touch with your whole hand, your partner feels the touch as an embrace, as if the touch were actually coming straight from your heart.

FIVE SIMPLE STROKES ARE ALL YOU NEED

You'll need only five basic strokes to give a sensuous massage: gliding, kneading, vibration, brush strokes and stillness.

Gliding
The first stroke you'll want to do is called gliding. Try it on yourself first, so that you'll see how it will feel to your partner. Place your hand on the back of your forearm, hearts of palms first. Let your fingers curl gently. Slowly pull your hand toward your shoulder, allowing your fingers to trail behind. The secret to gliding is to keep your hand relaxed. You can glide from your partner's shoulder all the way down to her toes and back again with one long stroke.

Don't lift your hands. Go s-l-o-w-l-y. No one ever com-
plains that a massage was done too slowly.

Kneading
Kneading is great to use to supplement your gliding strokes.
Knead with your palm and let your fingers follow. Use your
whole hand to squeeze and pull the muscle. Depending on
your intention, this stroke can feel deep and invigorating
or delicate and relaxing.

Vibration
A great way to get muscles to relax. Place your hands,
palm first, on your partner's body. Let your fingers relax.
With alternating side-to-side motions of your hands, be-
gin a slow vibration. Vibrations feel amazing on the but-
tocks. Play around—this can bring out the giggles in your
partner.

Brush Strokes
Using your fingertips, lightly stroke your lover's body (re-
member to stroke, not poke). The stroking can be done in
a circular or back-and-forth motion, or you can slowly
trace your way around their body.

Stillness
Your hands don't need to be in constant motion. We begin
and end every Bondassage session with stillness. A power-
ful way of connecting is to hold your hands on their body
and simply match your breathing to theirs. Stay present
and help your partner go deeper into pleasure.

These five simple strokes can be used in any combination and on any part of the body, including the genitals. For example, you could use brush strokes over your lover's penis, then slide your hands back and forth on either side of it, then hold your hands perfectly still as you keep him just this side of orgasm.

Generally, the order of a massage is: back, backs of arms, butt, legs and feet, then have your partner turn over. On the front, start at the top of the body and work your way down. Teasingly visit the genitals often—it's lovely to have one hand on the genitals while you're stroking another body part.

EROTIC BACK BODY MASSAGE

Start by connecting with your partner. Place your hands—one on the upper back at the heart and one on the sacrum—and breathe with them. Next, start slow, gentle rocking up and down the body to help them loosen up and drop deep into their body. Continue with slow, light, whole-hand glides down the body. In Bondassage, we like to use soft, silky items next. A satin pillowcase floated slowly over the body, rabbit fur mitts rubbed delightfully down the sides of the body, over the tush, between the toes and up the inner thighs. A feather duster, a string of pearls, cool links of chain ... use your imagination.

Back
Stand at the head of the table (or at their shoulder if you're shorter or they have headphones on). Put a little warmed oil in your hands and rub them together. Spread the warm oil slowly down their back, shoulders, neck and arms. Enjoy connecting with your partner in a relaxed way and just offer them pleasure.

Make small thumb circles down each side of the spine from the neck to the tailbone. Have your thumbs mirror each other as they circle outward from the spine. Vary this stroke by using your hands to glide down their back or from side to side across their body. See how slowly you can go.

Arms
Cupping your hands over the tops of your partner's arms, slide slowly down their arm, squeezing firmly, all the way down to the wrist in one continuous stroke. Repeat several times, experimenting with your own variations—glide softly, use brush strokes with your fingertips, or simply press and hold.

Lower Body
Kneeling in between your partner's legs, rest a hand on their lower back and pour a bit of warm oil into your palm. Rub your hands together. Keeping contact with the skin, spread the oil from the buttocks down the legs to the bottoms of their feet. Slowly and deeply massage the pads and the arches. Lightly run your hands up the insides of their legs, lingering over the sensitive inner thighs and back up over their buttocks. Repeat several times. Vary your stroke speed and intensity.

Tease the back of the knees and thighs with your fingertips or the back of your hand. It's delicious to come close to the genitals and then back away.

Finishing Massage Strokes On The Back Body

Say goodbye to the back of your partner's body with the same full-body glides you used to introduce the massage. Trace the whole body from head to foot in a long, continuous path. Finish by gently resting your hands over their heart and sacrum and breathe with your partner.

EROTIC FRONT BODY MASSAGE

Many of us have issues with our bodies, and being massaged on the front of the body can make us feel particularly vulnerable. Blindfolds can help relieve the receiver's self-consciousness for the receiver and we recommend them highly.

As the giver, begin by re-connecting with your partner. Place your hands—one at the heart and one on the genitals—and breathe with them. Continue with slow, light, whole-hand glides up and down the body. Use silky, soft, furry sensation play items next. Jaeleen loves to slowly drag her hot pink rabbit fur flogger up and down her partner's body, stopping at the soles of the feet to do some light flogging.

Upper Front Body

From a kneeling position between your partner's legs, rub warmed oil over their upper body, starting with the belly, coming up between the breasts with one hand following the other. At the collarbone, press outward toward the edges of the shoulders, then continue down the arms all the way to the fingertips, where you will lift gently off.

Abdomen

Using the palm of your hand, circle a gentle clockwise motion around the navel several times. Trace the ridge of the lower ribs with your fingertips. Finish by sliding both hands up the side body from the hips until you reach the underarms.

Shoulders/Arms/Hands

Place both palms on the upper chest, above the breasts, with your fingers pointing to 10 and 2. Slowly and firmly press outward toward the shoulder edges. Knead the upper shoulders and arms by squeezing the muscles, moving downward to the forearms and wrists. Squeeze the hand gently, roll each finger slowly between your thumb and first finger, and entwine your fingers with theirs.

Chest/Breast

Now it's time for a special treat. Men, as well as women, can enjoy sensual breast massage and erotic artists can draw out and prolong the pleasure of breast stimulation. Many people report feeling an electric "zing" from the nipples to the genitals.
Breast massage strokes will be covered in more depth in a later chapter.

Lower Front Body Massage

You have awakened your partner's body with silks, furs, or feathers. Now it's time to go deeper with your strokes. Sit between their legs, straddling the massage table if comfortable, and pull their knees over your thighs. Using warm oil, spread it slowly over the outside of the legs, down to the feet and trace back up the insides of the legs towards the genitals.

Legs

Massage her thighs, calves and feet. You can play with increasing and decreasing the sexual energy with the direction of your strokes. Going up the thighs toward the genitals increases the sexual energy. Moving your hands down the legs away from the genitals decreases and grounds the energy. Press your thumbs into the sole of the foot and knead in small circles. Slide a finger in and out between the toes, then gently grasp and squeeze the entire foot. A delightful little nibble may increase arousal here, (and other places as well).

Head

You may wish to have your partner's head in your lap for these strokes, or you may want to skip or modify this if part if they're wearing a blindfold and headphones.
Comb your fingers gently through their hair, gently tugging small sections. Using the pads of your fingers, firmly massage the scalp in small circles. With your thumbs, make small circles at the temples and behind her jaw.
Find the ridge where the skull meets the neck. Holding the weight of her head a couple of inches off your lap, knead this ridge using your fingertips.
Featherweight touch on the face, the eyes, the mouth, the ears can be terribly exciting. Dare to put your fingers in your lover's mouth and see if they suck, nibble, or lick. We're sure they will not be displeased.

Finishing Strokes For The Front Body

Place your hand over their heart. Think of penetrating your lover's heart with your caring, your protection and your love. You are in the bubble, and everything contained in the bubble is erotic connectivity. Brush your fingertips slowly over their body, from their head down to their toes. We will discuss more later on about specifics on how to caress the erogenous zones and bring your partner to orgasm. It's lovely to cover your lover with a blanket, tuck them in, and leave them to soak in the afterglow.

> *"First, a nice relaxing massage, followed by some truly wicked teasing and trance-like body percussion. It drove me crazy. Just thinking about it makes me wish I were on the table right now!"—Michael*

BOOBIE BLISS

"It's rare in today's world that we have a chance to completely surrender all of our responsibilities, thoughts, worries and concepts of ourselves and go inward. Exploring physical pleasure can leave you inspired. Playing with magical states of mind can provide a fresh outlook on life. Touch and human connection is food for your soul."—Audrey

As we've already stated, once your partner is blindfolded she will find that physical stimulation increases vastly. This can work well for you when it comes to nipple stimulation, or not so well, depending on the person. For some, nipple stimulation is hardly erotic at all—perhaps even a turn-off. On the other end of the spectrum are those who easily reach orgasm by nipple stimulation alone—like there's a live wire running directly from their nipples to their genitals. Some research also suggests men often become more receptive to nipple stimulation after the age of forty. Further, it is also possible to condition your partner's responsiveness by stimulating the nipples as she orgasms repeatedly. Of course, if your partner is completely uncomfortable with nipple play, you may need to keep it to feather light caresses and soft kisses. Once again, talking about it and then watching how she responds will work better than simply charging in with the clamps.

Some people prefer only the lightest of touches on their nipples; others love strong pinches and bites. Some love the spectrum. If you play with such stimulation, always start slowly and lightly and build up gradually to the stronger stuff, particularly if this is a new partner. Of course, like beautiful music, you will want to change the rhythm and cadence of the song you are playing. Many people, especially women, find that their breasts respond to lengthy overtures of stroking and kissing.

After you have massaged your partner and flipped her over onto her back, the breasts are all yours. Some like constant stimulation, (nipple clamps and suction work well here to leave your hands for other devices), others like pauses.

For a fun variation, you can wrap the erect part of the nipple firmly with dental floss. This will cause the tip of the nipple to become highly sensitive. Gently lick, brush feathers, or use ice to play with the sensations. Use lots of wraps so that the floss doesn't cut into the tender tissue of the nipple and finish it with a bow for easy removal. What a gift!

Kneeling between her legs or sitting at her side, add warmed oil to your hands and, cupping a hand around each breast, vibrate the fleshy tissue. Imagine telling your partner how beautiful her breasts are and how much pleasure it brings you to touch them. Most women think they are too big, too small, or too something. Support her surrender in this vulnerable area with your deep breathing and conscious touch.

With both hands on one breast, encircle the entire breast, gently pulling up on it and squeezing. Take the time to feel its silky texture and softness. Repeat these movements on the other breast.

Experiment with tracing patterns such as a spirals and circles in towards the nipple and back out. Use a light touch at first.

Ready to play with the nipples yet? Use your thumb to barely brush over the oiled tip of the nipple. Pause. Teasingly flick the nipple with your thumb. Stop. Silence is a stroke. Roll the nipple with your thumb and index finger. Err on the side of too little, not too much.

Come in to where she can feel your hot breath just hanging over the nipple. Breathe several deep breaths without touching, just breath on skin. If you leave her wanting more, you've done your job.

Strokes to try:

Spirals
With your fingertip circling the outer part of your lover's breast, delicately and slowly trace a spiral inwardly. Eventually your finger will spiral up to the nipple. Or try rubbing the nipples with the inside of your forearm.

Liftoff
Squeeze the base of the nipple between the pads of your index finger and thumb. Then slide up and off the nipple, alternating your hands, one immediately after the other.

Oral Strokes
Encircle your lips around the areola. If the suction is with the lips only, the sensation is good—however it is truly exquisite when the nipple is farther inside the mouth between the tongue and upper palate. There's a secret to this:

Never entirely release your suction. The nipple moves back and forth, but always keep at least a minimal suction.

For an epicurean variation, gently spread whipped cream or honey over your lover's breast, then savor.

Nipple Strokes

Caress his cock and balls with one of your nipples. Or try caressing his nipples with one of yours.

PUSSY PLEASURING

"Pleasure is your birthright."—Dreu

Female genital massage is a sensuous form of bodywork that can build trust between lovers. It helps her connect to her inner sensuality and results in feelings of complete well-being, satisfaction and contentment. The genitals are sensitive but they are by no means delicate—we don't need to treat them with kid gloves (unless you're into that sort of thing).

A woman loves to have her pussy honored and adored, and treated with respect. There are many exquisite parts to touch, explore and appreciate. Glide with your fingertips over her clitoris, between the labia, gently pull on her labial lips, press your hand over her vulva, touch slowly, even more slowly, stop and let your touch be still.

The tissue of the inner labia and the vagina is mucous membrane, the same type of tissue that is inside the eyelid, so make sure these tissues are kept moist and touched with care. Part of this care includes short and smooth fingernails with the skin beside the nails also filed smooth.

Use body strokes to spread the sexual energy from the

genitals, stroking from the pussy to the belly and heart, and from the genitals or heart out to the arms and legs. Beginning at the pussy or the heart, stroke down each of the legs and up each of the arms, making a large U-shape. Spread the energy throughout the massage as well, as you want to bring your partner back from the edge.

When you are both ready to begin the massage, have her lie on her back (headphones on and blindfolded) with one pillow under her head and another under her hips to elevate her pelvis. Ask her to bend her knees and open her legs to expose her genitals. You can either sit comfortably between her legs with your legs crossed, or you may wish to straddle the table (if you're using a massage table) and drape her open legs over yours.

Place your hands at the outer tops of her thighs and hold for a moment. Watch her breathing and connect with her. Connect her heart to her vulva by placing one hand on her heart space between her breasts and the other hand, lightly and softly cupped against her vulva. Hold this position for several breaths, using this time to feel in your body, to notice her breathing, and to let her feel the heart/genital connection. Feel the connection between the two of you through your touch and presence.

Gently massage the legs, abdomen and thighs to encourage her to relax. Next, massage the pubic bone area and then move down to the inner thigh area. Gently draw your fingertips up along the inner thighs and vaginal lips. Tug gently on her pubic hair. Always remember to have a slow hand and an easy touch.

Pour a small quantity of warm, high-quality oil or lubricant on her pubic mound. Coconut oil is a favorite—it has antibacterial properties and smells wonderful. Pour just enough so that it drips down the outer lips and covers the outside of the genitals. Begin gently massaging the mound and outer lips. Slowly and sensually massage her outer lips. With the thumb and index finger, gently squeeze each lip, sliding the fingers up and down the entire length. Carefully repeat this process with each inner lip of the vagina varying the pressure and speed of touch based on what feels right. Spend time here and do not rush.

The clitoris is an amazingly complex structure, similar in function to the penis, but many times more sensitive. The glans portion of the clitoris holds more sensory nerve endings than any other structure in the human body. The clitoris has only one purpose: pleasure. Nothing tops its ability to receive and transmit sensations of touch, pressure or vibration.

Gently stroke the clitoris in a circular motion, clockwise and counter-clockwise. Lightly squeeze it between thumb and index fingers. Many women report that it feels better when you lick or caress the sides of her clitoris rather than its top. You can use your other hand to massage her breasts, abdomen, or inner thighs.

Move on to teasing the outside of the vaginal opening after you've done a nice warm-up massage of the whole area. Tease along the outside of the vaginal opening and around, near the outside of the vaginal opening just above, to the urethra. The urethra also has erectile tissue in it which can also be a source of great pleasure. Many women like having their urethra stimulated very lightly while lubricated. We, of course, suggest trying it to find out.

As you move to the vaginal opening make sure not to penetrate right away. It is crucial to proceed very slowly with internal touch in order to let your partner relax. Take time around that opening to tease, to massage, to allow her to draw you inside.

Next, slowly insert your middle finger into her. Very gently explore and massage the inside with your finger. Take your time and gently feel up, down and sideways. Due to differences in pelvic structures, the G-spot might actually be anywhere from just an inch above the pubic bone (near 12:00) to somewhere near the uterus. With your palm pointing upward and your finger inside your partner's pussy, bend your finger to make contact with her G-spot. Gentle pressure from the other hand can be added on the lower abdomen just above the pubic bone.

Be gentle and take your time. If a single finger is well received, you may be able to increase the pleasure by the addition of another. Try using the thumb of your hand to stimulate the clitoris. If you're feeling adventurous, and she seems open to it, you might try inserting the pinky of the right hand into her anus.

Enjoy giving the massage without any expectations. Support your partner in having the type of finish that she would like, whether it is to have a climax through her own touch, through your touch, with a vibrator or toys, or to retain the energy through the clench and hold:

The clench and hold is a tantric practice: Instruct the recipient to start with deep breathing through her mouth. Once she feels tingly and alive (at least thirty breaths or so), she should take three fast deep breaths, then clenches her PC muscles (the pelvic floor muscles that keep you from peeing), and the muscles through her entire body, holding her breath for as long as she can. You may then tell her to release and feel the flood of sensations!

As she comes back to earth, place one hand on her heart and one hand on her genitals and take some nice deep breaths together. Slowly, gently, and with respect, remove your hands. Cover her genitals with warm, wet towels and wrap her in a blanket. Allow her to relax and enjoy the afterglow.

PENIS PLEASURING

The combination of virtuoso massage skills, "body percussion," sensation play and sensory deprivation was like nothing I'd ever experienced. I was taken right to the edge then back again."—Sebastien

A man loves to have his penis and balls played with, tickled, fondled, massaged and worshipped. Slowly and gradually appreciate and explore every square inch of his genital surface area. Let your fingers flow from the balls to the top of the cock, swirl around the head, then slide back down the other half and end back down at the balls. Make him feel your intention to fully explore his beautiful cock.

If you know your partner is a "quick shot," make most of your strokes light and mostly away from the tip until you are ready to allow him to release. Make use of anal stimulation and the many ball and scrotum strokes. To bring your partner back from the edge, place your hands on the pelvis and stroke down the legs and off the feet, several times if necessary, until he calms down.

Use body strokes to spread the sexual energy from the

genitals, stroking from his cock to the belly and heart, and from the genitals or heart out to the arms and legs. Spread the energy throughout the massage as well, as you want to bring your partner back from the edge.

If you're looking for an easy and effective way to spice up masturbating him, simply drape a bed sheet on top of his penis as you're stroking it. Satin, bamboo or fleece sheets offer an extra-sensual variation.

Have your lover lie on his back, headphones on and blindfolded, with a pillow under his head.

Place a pillow, covered with a towel, underneath his butt. His legs should be spread apart with the knees slightly bent (pillows or cushions under the knees will also help) and his genitals clearly exposed for the massage. You can either sit comfortably between his legs with your legs crossed, or you may wish to straddle the table (if you're using a massage table) and drape his open legs over yours

Place your hands at the outer tops of his thighs and hold for a moment. Watch his breathing, and connect with him. Connect his heart to his cock by placing one hand on his heart space in the center of his chest and the other hand, lightly and softly cupped, against his cock. Hold this position for several breaths, using this time to feel in your body, to notice his breathing, and to let him feel the heart/genital connection. Feel the connection between the two of you through your touch and presence.

Place your non-dominant hand a few inches over your lover's genitals, palm down, and your fingers slightly separated. Pour the heated massage oil over the back of this hand. Let the warm oil drips between your fingers onto the penis and scrotum. Use a generous amount of oil, and with loving strokes, spread it slowly and completely over all of his genital area.

Olive or coconut oil can make an excellent lubricant for erotic massage. It's cheap, tastes wonderful and maintains a good slickness. However, like all oils, it's not latex-friendly, so reserve it for times when there is no latex nearby.

Rub the oil into his skin, starting off at the very top the inner thighs and sliding slowly into the crease where his legs meet the pelvic floor. Using unhurried, steady motions, work along the connecting bone and muscles, soothing tension as you go.

The following massage techniques aren't intended to get your man off as quickly as possible—quite the opposite! Bondassage is all about tease and denial.

Use various tempos and pressures and change them often. Alternate high-energy strokes with slower ones. Alternate strokes that concentrate on the glans with strokes that totally focus on the shaft. Mix it up—keep him guessing!

Don't forget the body strokes. Spread that sexual energy up from his cock, into his belly and heart, and out to his arms and legs.

Wake It Up
Begin by kneading and lightly scratching the pubic mound. Stroke, tickle and tug gently on the hair of the scrotum. If the skin of the scrotum is fairly loose, you can knead it (not the testicles themselves, only the scrotal skin). The sides and rear wall of the scrotum are often tremendously sensitive to light stroking by fingers or tongue.

Ball Pulls
Try a gentle ball pull—encircle the top of his scrotum with your thumb and forefinger. Squeeze this ring together until it's snug and his testicles are "trapped" below it. Slowly

and gently pull down so that the skin of his scrotum is pulled tight over his testicles. Lightly pull just a bit more for about five seconds while you proceed to pleasure his cock, then release the pull (but keep your hand in place). Closely watch his face, breathing and body for his response. Repeat, varying the intensity and duration of the pull while you combine it with more pleasure on his cock. Once you have his balls "trapped," you'll be able to stroke and lightly scratch the firmly stretched skin over them to excellent effect.

The Root

The shaft extends farther back into the body. Discovering and stimulating the hidden areas of the shaft provides an unaccustomed, impressive, enjoyable sensation for him. Position your fingers in the area in back of his scrotum, and press up. You'll be able to feel the part of the shaft you can't see. When you've got it between your fingers, slide back and forth. Expand your stroke to include the perineum, another ignored portion of the male anatomy (the perineum is the section of tissue between the scrotum and the anus and it's rich in nerve endings). This specific stroke hits nerves from the area around the prostate gland and carries sensations right down to the tip of the penis. You may need extra lube for the longer strokes, so have some nearby.

Lift-off

One stroke that Jaeleen finds really effective is this one: While you massage the shaft, gently but firmly squeeze his cock at the base with your right hand and pull up, sliding completely off the top. Then do the same motion using your left hand—squeeze his cock at the base and pull up, sliding completely off. Do this again with your right, then your left, and so on. Eventually change directions—slide alternating hands from the top down to the base. Use both hands alternately to rub in a downward direction, so he'll feel as if he's just going deeper and deeper and deeper inside you and then change directions.

Firestarter

Take his cock in between both hands and rub your hands rapidly back and forth, as if you wanted to start a fire. Grasp his cock by the head and gently shake it back and forth. Thoroughly massage the head by cupping it in your palm and turning your wrist, making "juicing" motion (as if you are juicing a lemon). The spot on the underside of the penis, just slightly below the notch in the head, is extremely responsive to being licked and stroked. Shift from his cock to the testicles to the perineum and back again, observing his responses.

Climbing The Mountain

Take his cock in one hand and gently, sensuously caress it for around ten seconds, then give it one quick up-and-down stroke. Repeat the sensuous caressing for about 10 seconds, perhaps doing slow up-and-down strokes, perhaps doing other things that feel great to him, then give his penis 2 quick up-and-down strokes. Repeat the sensual caressing, then give 3 quick strokes. Then more caressing, followed by 4 quick strokes. Then more caressing, and 5 strokes. Continue to "climb the mountain" as long as you both can stand it.

Breath Work

If you gently blow on something like a penis or nipple from very close, your breath appears to be warm. If you back off about 6-12 inches and blow, your breath feels deliciously cool. Wetting the blown-upon object using your saliva boosts both the sensations. Cold and hot can be alternated to incredible effect.

Some men have trouble reaching orgasm if their legs are spread apart. Having him bound with his legs spread wide will allow you to prolong the tease and denial session enormously.

Enjoy the massage without any expectations. Support your partner in having the type of finish to the session that he would like, whether it is to have a climax through your touch, through his touch, through a combination of your touch and his, with a vibrator or any toys, or to retain the energy through the male-bodied version of the clench and hold:

Instruct him to start with deep breathing through his mouth. Once he feels tingly and alive (at least thirty breaths or so), have him take three fast deep breaths, then clenches his PC muscles (the pelvic floor muscles), and the muscles through his entire body, holding his breath for as long as he can. Then have him release and feel the flood of sensations!

If he decides to ejaculate, don't stop stroking him as soon as all of the ejaculate is gone. Keep going until the orgasm stops. You can often provide him a small "extra" orgasm by pinching his cock lightly but securely and "milking" the residual fluid from his penis after his "regular" orgasm has finished. You can also place your thumb at the base of his cock and your finger at the rear top of his scrotum and milk that section forward, then bring your hand forward and milk the penis from base to tip, providing a more thorough draining.

BOOTY BACCHANALIA

"It's a relaxing exploration with a combination of new & familiar sensations. I entered a cocoon of darkness, music and warmth, an oasis where I gently let go of control and surrendered to pure bliss."—Jo

The receiving partner should tell their lover about their past experiences (or lack thereof) regarding anal sex, particularly any problems that have occurred. They should also mention any anal or rectal problems they have, such as hemorrhoids, fissures, an enlarged prostate, or more serious medical conditions. Those with heart problems should be aware that heavy bearing down, during anal play or during a bowel movement, can slow the speed and force of their heartbeat, occasionally to zero. Use appropriate caution and get a medical consultation as necessary.

If you are the receiver, it is up to you how clean you would like to be as well as how much time you have to prepare. If you have plenty of time, don't eat for at least 12 hours prior. 4-6 hours prior, get an enema bag and give yourself an enema. Use a minimum of 1 quart and up to 2 quarts of warm (105-108 degrees) water with 1 teaspoon salt per quart. Retain each enema for 10-15 minutes, repeat until the entire enema appears clear, usually 3-4 times, more if you can't take the minimum of a full quart. If you've got a colon tube, you can use that also, and that will clean you *all* the way up.

If you have never done an enema, try doing one a week or so before instead of the day of play to discover how it feels, in addition to just how long it takes you to feel prepared. It'll also let you discover how your body responds to enemas. If you feel light-headed following the enemas, increase the salt to 1 ½ teaspoons per quart of water, as multiple enemas can dehydrate you.

For a quick clean of only the important parts in a pinch, use a lube shooter (available from any sex toy store or website), fill it full of a water-based lube and inject. You should have a bowel movement within 15-30 minutes. Follow that with another lube shooter and you will be good to go. This will only clean out the last 6-12 inches, but is usually ok in an emergency. As a bonus, you'll be pre-lubed for whatever comes up (or goes in).

The anal region contains a good number of nerve endings and can be a place of great relaxation and great pleasure. Both external and internal touch can be extremely relaxing and arousing. There is no rush to "get in the door," so really linger doing external touch. Slow exquisite touch can take your partner to states perhaps previously unknown, both in terms of relaxation and arousal. Reports of orgasm from anal play alone are not rare. Still, this activity shouldn't be done hurriedly or carelessly.

Lots of lube is another key for anal play. The vagina and the mouth supply their own lubrication: the rectum doesn't. While the vagina often needs extra lubrication, the rectum always does. Generally speaking, heavier, more gel-like lubricants will usually perform better than lighter, more liquid ones. Nowadays, water-soluble lubricants are preferred over oil-soluble lubricants, especially when latex condoms and/or gloves are used. Avoid colored or scented lubricants. Remember: "Lube early, lube often."

Disease can be transmitted in both directions during anal play. Because of this, we strongly recommend barrier usage even for partners who don't use condoms for or barriers for other kinds of sex. Dildos, plugs, vibrators and penises should be covered with condoms. Fingers and hands should be covered with gloves. Toys and hands should be cleaned afterwards.

While erotic fiction contains many depictions of a person hating yet loving having something shoved suddenly and deeply into their rectum by an uncaring, dominant partner, the truth is far different. Doing this may cause them serious injury, and they most likely will hate it.

The anus has two rings of sphincter muscle: the external and the internal. The outer sphincter muscle is that cute little pucker between your partner's cheeks. The internal sphincter takes longer to release. Going slow is the key. If you think you are going slow, go even slower! The anus is a place where a lot of tension and emotion is stored, so going slowly allows the muscles to relax. Never push in. A relaxed muscle can stretch—a tight muscle is rigid and can rip. Relaxed muscles can feel more, as well. Use your slow touch to allow your partner to relax and feel more!

As your partner relaxes, the anus will draw you in. Again, linger with your external touch, for relaxation and pleasure. Pressure on the rosebud, with no intent to enter, can be very relaxing and arousing. A still, holding touch can be more powerful than even the most vigorous stimulation, so—go slow.

Start very gently and, wearing a glove or finger cot (placing a cotton ball in the fingertip of your glove can help eliminate any "sharp" feeling, particularly if you have long fingernails), trace the outside very gently using your ring finger.

Begin by slowly spreading the butt cheeks with both hands. Place your thumbs on each side of the anus. Pressing down gently, pull your thumbs gradually apart. Watching your partner's breathing, stretch with their inhalation, return with their exhalation. Inch your thumbs to more of a diagonal position around the anus and pull diagonally. Inch your thumbs above and below and pull up and down. Doing these gentle stretches with the breath is key.

Rest one hand between the butt cheeks so the tip of your index finger is touching the anus, then rest your other hand on the sacrum. Keeping both hands soft, lightly press and release on the anus in time with their breathing. Slowly press around the anus, imagining that it's a clock. Start at 12:00 and continue clockwise, stopping to press for a few seconds at each "hour."

Using plenty of lube, rest one finger on the anus and, very gently, apply pressure allowing them to draw you in. *Do not push in.* Hold still for at least 30 seconds once you're inside the first sphincter (one knuckle). Pay close attention. You might feel fluttering light spasms or twitches in the first two inches of the canal. Remain motionless for a couple of minutes. As your partner relaxes, you can begin to slowly insert your finger deeper. With your palm facing the front of your partner's body, start a gentle "come-here" motion. Gently explore the front, side and back walls. Move your finger like a windshield wiper over the front inner wall. Trace circles and figure-eights, alternating the speed, depth and pressure of your stroke.

When you are able to move one finger in and out easily, add additional lube and try slowly inserting a second finger. We highly recommend you don't insert a vibrator or dildo until you can easily move two fingers completely in and out. Having this done to you personally will teach you quite a bit about how precisely to do it to someone else.

Successful anal penetration requires feedback. Just a small variation in pressure, location, depth, or angle often makes a huge difference in how well the play goes. The receiving partner must communicate these matters clearly and promptly to the inserting person so necessary adjustments can be made. Above all, the receiving partner shouldn't "tough it out" in silence in an effort to please their lover. If something feels wrong, it almost undoubtedly is wrong and it needs prompt correction. Anal play is not the time for the receptive partner to take a "stoic heroic" approach. Ongoing communication and adjustment are essential.

Many heterosexual guys are intrigued by the thought of anal play, but have been given a number of erroneous ideas that anal play is somehow the exclusive province of gay men. Nothing could be further from the truth. Every man has a prostate gland, and quite a few men, straight and gay alike, find stimulation of the prostate to be sexually arousing—nothing about anal play is inherently "gay" (unless, of course, you're doing it with another man). If you've been avoiding this nerve-rich and exciting part of your body on account of something someone suggested years ago, you've got a treat in store.

The initial entry of anal insertion is often the most uncomfortable part for the receptive partner. This discomfort can often be minimized by holding the plug or dildo stationary and letting him "back" onto it at his own pace. Entry can be made more comfortable if he bears down (as he does when having a bowel movement) as the object is being inserted. Lovers who enjoy using butt plugs on themselves often set the plug down, business end up, on a chair or toilet seat cover and gradually lower themselves onto it.

If he's a novice to the sensations of anal sex, you may be finding it hard to tell which sensations are "right" and which ones mean something's wrong. Generally, mild sensations of stretching, pain and burning and feelings of having to defecate are normal, especially at first. Any sharp pain, intense burning, or pain that lasts past the first couple of minutes will be a sign that something isn't right. Almost everyone has an instinctive sense of the distinction between "good pain" and bad pain"—if he's feeling the second one, stop, ease off, try a smaller insertable or more lubrication or maybe more relaxation, or just move to another activity and try again another time. Being goal-oriented isn't a good strategy during any type of sex, but most especially during anal sex.

Finally, make sure you remove your anal toy slowly and carefully. Yanking it out feels unpleasant and can cause injury. Ask your partner to push or bear down at the count of three. That way, you both work together in finalizing the scene.

HIDDEN TREASURES

*"I am always a bit nervous exploring
things on the edge but my lover made
it safe, hot and fun."—Deanna*

A good massage can be relaxing or invigorating, but it is not necessarily erotic. In Bondassage, we like to make the mundane sexy and keep it that way. Knowing your partner and all their various turn-ons will help determine how to augment their arousal. And then of course, there are verified tricks to increasing arousal starting with erogenous zones.

THE EROGENOUS ZONES

Intense, prolonged arousal is a win/win for everybody. The giver gets to take the receiver on an amazing erotic journey and the receiver gets to fly. In order to move from the sensuous to the erotic, (sensual), you'll want to stimulate specific points on the body with the intention of building that amazingly intense, prolonged arousal. You can use the prolonged arousal to build the erotic aspects of your play, bringing your partner to edge over and again. You may wish to even use a safe word here to allow your partner to indicate their desire for orgasm so that you may control it better. Knowing where to go to continue the pace without stopping will help you do just that.

There are three main groups of erogenous zones on the body:

Primary Erogenous Zones
The first set of primary zones are the most potent of the bunch. You will want to manipulate them sparingly until you get to know the effects:

mouth
breast and nipples
genitals

Secondary Erogenous Zones
The secondary zones are those we classically think of when we consider the less-than-obvious areas that are still "sexy":

earlobes
nape of the neck
inside of the thigh
base of the spine
space where the buttock meets the top of the thigh

Tertiary Erogenous Zones
The third tier of zones are less than obvious, but can help you continue the erotic stimulation without necessarily going too far. Please note however, that with extended play, some people can find themselves orgasmic from secondary or tertiary stimulation:

outside surface of the little finger
center of the palm
nostrils
ear canal
sole of the foot
big toe
back of the knee
navel
anus

To steadily increase arousal, start with the second or third zones then move in toward the first. Alternate your movements to increase and decrease arousal to suit you and your partner's desires. For example, you can begin by biting the nape of the neck, then kissing a nipple. Move down the body with a 2-handed, whole-hand-touching, gliding stroke until you reach the foot. Kiss the foot or nibble on the big toe, then lick your way up the leg to the back of the knee, where you can smooch and lick. Follow up with a teasing deep kiss on the mouth. Your partner should be moaning with delight.

Some other erogenous zones are: the mouth (why is kissing so erotic?), the scalp (oooh, the feeling of a light head rub!), the neck (did you say nibble?), and the ears (oooh, more nibbling!).

The chest and nipples are often an extreme erogenous zone, especially for women. The abdomen and navel are also quite sensual, provided your partner will let you. Many people feel uncomfortable having their navels touched. The tailbone has all kinds of nerve endings. Lightly rub your partner's tailbone and watch their tail wag!

Our arms love touch also: note the inside of the elbow and

forearm and how wonderful it feels to be stroked. Another "taboo" area is the underarm, chocked full of pheromones (see scent), they are also excellent sources of pleasant erotic touch. Of course, fingers also love being touched (what a novelty!), and the insides of the fingers can be quite a sensual delight.

Like the arms, behind the knees are a wonderful erogenous zone on the legs, and, lest we forget, that lovely thigh area moving towards the genitals. Of course feet and toes have historically been erogenous zones for thousands of years. Some people claim to be able to orgasm simply from touch, and feet are high on the list of those areas.

The preferred desire is to drive your partner wild with pleasure, not to follow a pattern to the letter. Becoming aware of where the zones are and the pleasure your partner experiences when you move from one to another will help you take them there. You will soon see your partner reach intense new levels of arousal. In fact, you may actually see waves of pleasure rippling through the body in the form of sweet muscle twitches, vibrations and shakes. At the end of your play, your partner will be reinvigorated and grateful for the energetic releases you helped give them, even if they do not understand that is what has occurred.

Knowing erogenous zones and how to excite them will help create intense prolonged orgasmic bliss. Although the most common way to stimulate the body is with your hands and mouth, there are an infinite number of other ways to provide pleasure. Combining and alternating harder and softer touches keeps your partner alive, alert and turned on. Sensation-creating devices can be found throughout your house, (feather dusters, spoons, furry gloves, perfume, etc), as well as in sex shops and on the internet. Once you feel comfortable using your hands, mouth and other parts of your body, you can begin exploring erogenous zones using the vast array of materials at your fingertips.

CLENCH AND HOLD

We've described this remarkable technique elsewhere, but it bears repeating: as the recipient, start with deep breathing through your mouth. Keep breathing, enjoying the sensations in your body. Once you feel tingly and alive (at least thirty breaths or so), take three fast deep breaths, then clench your PC muscles, (the pelvic floor muscles that keep you from peeing), and tense the muscles through your entire body, holding your breath for as long as you can. Release and feel the flood of sensations!

EDGING

Another wonderful way of connecting with your partner is to "control" their orgasm. This can be done in several ways, but the basic technique is to bring your partner to the brink of orgasm, (many people think they know their partner's body really well, but even still this exercise is best verbal), and when she feels ready to explode, she must ask for permission to "release." Of course, if that feels too demanding or controlling, you can also use a safe word like "yellow." You can then slow down or stop the massage strokes, bringing them down, only to bring them up again. This technique is also called "edging" and can help your partner have an incredibly explosive orgasm! What a great way to make an intimate connection.

TOOLS & TECHNIQUES

"Next comes the spice! A little bit of this a little bit of that and delicious edges of soft and hard pleasure. Weaving together massage with light BDSM this is a treat for the senses that is not to be missed!"—Anya

Before getting started in your Bondassage play, you will need a few items to get you ready. We already introduced you to the basics in chapter one, but here is a more complete list of everything that might go into your Bondassage kit. Once you've grown more comfortable with the equipment and techniques, you may wish to start adding more. We suggest you go through the list and determine your comfort level; not everything is necessary to start, but you will want to at least have a means for lying down, some type of restraint, blindfold, music, massage cream and a few toys.

BONDASSAGE SUPPLY LIST

General Equipment

Massage Table. We converted ours to bondage tables by drilling holes down each side at about 8" intervals and installing eye bolts, but you can start with any sturdy massage table.

Flat black satin (or otherwise) sheets. Full size if you plan on wrapping your partner in the sheet at the end, or twin if you plan to use a blanket.

Standard size pillow with satin pillow case.

Black jersey pillow case for the face cradle.

Blanket.

Bolster (optional but nice).

1 small towel.

2 hot wet towels (heat in a plastic bag in the microwave).

Thermal-style case or towels/hot packs (optional).

Dual purpose massage cream.

Vitamin E oil/coconut oil.

Small Condoms for toys.

Finger Cots.

Latex gloves.

Water-based lube.

Moist towelettes.

Tissues.

Candles/lighter.

Bondage Equipment

Leather collar.

Wrist/Ankle cuffs (We use fur-lined leather ones).

Blindfold (also fur-lined or raised such as the Mindfold).
Music source—stereo/Mp3 player/computer hooked up to
speakers, loaded with appropriate music.
Wireless headphones used with a splitter that connects to
your speakers.
Cotton clothes line or 5/8" nylon rope (from the hardware
store or www.rainbowrope.com) 5 - 7' long pieces.

USING YOUR TOYS

Blindfolds

Decent inexpensive blindfolds, marketed as "sleep shades," can be bought at drugstores although travel shops carry better ones. Eve's favorite is the meditative blindfold, The Mindfold. Lightweight and comfortable, it is made to allow you to keep your eyes open while wearing it, wonderful! Remember, some people don't realize how claustrophobic they are until you put the blindfold on. Be open and compassionate if your partner doesn't like it, perhaps trying a light silk scarf gently placed over the eyes to start.

Clips and clamps

Ordinary spring-loaded wooden clothespins offer an excellent "getting started in SM " toy (tiny arts and craft ones are available, too). They are cheap, widely available and relatively "novice proof." For starters, we suggest that you purchase a small bag of them—a dozen or so. Try them on yourself first, even if you're more dominant than submissive in your desires. Apply the clothespins to dry skin, using dry fingers—you don't want them slipping off at the wrong moment. If the bite is too strong, try pulling its jaws apart to loosen it a bit. Start slowly and lightly. Gauging how much your partner likes nipple play will usually help you determine how much pressure they can take with clothespins or clamps.

If you find clothespins erotic for nipple play, you may want to invest in some clover clamps. These are a specific type of nipple clamp consisting of a clamp with a lever mechanism to which a chain or cord is affixed in such a way that pulling on the chain or cord increases pressure on the clamp.

Keep in mind that, unlike a swat from a hand or paddle, clamps may continue to hurt or the area may grow "numb." Of course, after you take them off the nipples will peak with a surge of immediate extreme sensation when the blood rushes back to the area. Unless you've experienced this yourself, you can easily forget that.

Vibrators

There are many vibrators from which to choose. Eve really likes the Hitachi Magic Wand since it is very strong (you can soften the intensity with a sock or rubber covering), has attachable insertables, and can be used as an actual massager, (that's what it's made for, hey). Of course, some people find it too strong or noisy, in which case, there are many lovely quieter models, particularly those made by Lelo, but you should be able to find a large selection at any online toy store like Good Vibrations or Babeland.

Anal Play

As sex educator Tristan Taromino says, "It's the great equalizer." All people have asses, and all asses can be erogenous zones. Many people get a little squicked by the idea of having that dirty place touched, so to help the psychology of your partner you might take a shower together beforehand. Some people may even take an enema before play. In either case, know that the area outside your anus, the outer sphincter and perineum, is quite safe for play even with your mouth and most certainly with gloved hands.

Start by massaging the anus and the perineum on the outside of the body. As the giver, have your receiving partner breathe and relax as you continue to massage the area. You may also want to use a vibrator, (with condom for hygiene, less mess) to help your partner relax more. Don't forget the sphincter is a muscle surrounded by some of the largest muscles in the body. The more relaxed the muscles are, the easier the play. When ready, gently insert a well-lubricated finger (with cot or glove) about two inches into the anus and gently continue the massage. You may even find an area that feels round and hard, just behind the pelvis. In men it is called the prostate, and it can be pleasurable to have the prostate massaged in circular motions all around the area. In women, you may find a similar area a little farther in, and it is commonly called the g-spot. The come hither motion, (fingers pushing up and towards you as she is on her back), is generally the most preferred. As always, enjoy yourself and go slowly. See the Booty Bacchanalia chapter for more anal play information.

Insertables

After you have massaged the genital and ass area a bit, you may wish to be a little more hands-free so you can continue to stimulate your partner. Butt plugs and vibrators are terrific tools for helping you expand your play. Gently begin to insert the lubed, covered plug or vibrator in the anus or vagina. Eve's favorite plug for men is the Aneros (not bad for women either), since it was designed by a Doctor to help strengthen the prostate. The Betty Dodson Vaginal Barbell is great for vaginal play and for ass play for all genders as well. And for the more adventuresome, the N'Joy line carries a vast array of stainless steel insertables that have a pleasing heft to them.

Many butt plugs have the nasty habit, with only the slightest encouragement from a cough or contraction, of making rather dramatic projectile exits (the Aneros stays in well). Consider the following solution: acquire 2 strips of 1 inch leather or heavy but soft, fabric, as long as needed. Tie one around your partner's waist. Split the second one down the middle halfway so it forms a "y" shape. Tie the unsplit end to the back so it acts as a thong/g-string resting in the crack of the buttocks covering the anus, thus holding the plug in. The "y" section can then part and go around the genitals, with each end tied to one side of the waist strap in front, leaving their genitals free for further machinations.

More toys you might like to use include:

> *Nipple suction cups (Jaeleen uses the rubber snake bite ones) or tweezer-style nipple clips.*
> *Disposable electric toothbrushes (for zippy scratchy fun!).*
> *Cane (see chapter on Paddles, Floggers and Crops, Oh My!).*
> *Flogger, (a fluffy "whip")—one larger leather/suede one and one small rabbit fur one.*
> *Wooden hair brush (for light paddling).*
> *Plastic hair pick with a pointy end.*
> *Fur mitts (for sensual play).*
> *Feathers (more sensual play).*

Wartenberg wheel (a stainless wheel used to tickle and prick the skin).

You should now have a better idea on how to get started with your Bondassage play. With tools in hand and techniques in mind, let's move on to...

A FEAST OF THE SENSES

*"Bondassage is genuinely a treat for me
to share with my partner. I love the vivid
buffet of experience that it offers. I integrate
my own ideas and inspirations during
play and feel like I'm orchestrating a truly
beautiful voyage for my lover."—Greta*

SIGHT, SOUND, TASTE, SMELL, TOUCH

Our senses act like instruments in an orchestra: sometimes they need to be played solo, often adding more instruments until we reach that magical crescendo of orgasmic bliss!

Removing certain senses can magnify the power of other senses.

In Bondassage we like to remove the receiver's sense of sight by use of a blindfold, and their ability to touch through gentle restraint, so that hearing, tasting, smell and the sense of being touched are highlighted. Sexual arousal, passion and lusty, juicy attraction are natural. The sights, the sounds, the smells, the tastes, and a lover's touch can all contribute to sexual turn-on.

SIGHT

Many people get alarmed when they see the words "sensory deprivation." They think of isolation tanks or other scary machines. The fact is, it's not all that scary and you can "deprive" yourself of a sense like eyesight simply by closing your eyes. Sensory deprivation means merely that you are removing one or more of the senses: sight, sound, smell, touch and taste. By doing so, you can heighten the other senses. Sight is the most effective one. When your partner can't see, their sense of touch is dramatically increased, along with their imagination.

Try this: touch your forearm while looking at at. How does it feel? Now, close your eyes and touch your forearm. How does that feel? Now imagine feeling that more intensely because you are being touched by another! Speaking of feeling sensation more intensely—exaggerating the input can also create sensory overload. In a Bondassage session, you will want to create the rhythm of the dance that involves an opus of deprivation and overload to help your partner dance and fly in extreme states of ecstasy.

Note: Not all senses are created equal. For example, if your partner blindfolds you and puts earplugs in your ears, your sense of taste may become exquisitely acute. Placing your partner in bondage may greatly heighten their ability to sense movement within the body.

Further, by depriving your partner of sight, hearing and speech, you are releasing them from sexual responsibility. Ensuring a sensory deprivation experience with the noise, sight and weight of the world lifted from the bound-one's shoulders, they are able to float free in the eroticism of the scene, secure in the knowledge they are looked after by their partner.

Let's examine some ways you can create a safe and nurturing environment for your partner by deliberately decreasing and increasing sensory input.

SOUND

Music helps your partner relax and fall into the beat. It also helps you move your body in rhythm so that you and your partner are in sync with the atmosphere. We love playing sultry ambient music with Bondassage, usually with no lyrics that are easily decipherable. We want our partner to groove, not think!

Some of Our Favorite Music for Bondassage:

Blues Au Feminin
Buddha-Bar VII
Buddha-Bar IX
Buddha Café 2
Buddha Lounge
Buddha Lounge 2
Buddha Lounge 5
Buddha Lounge 6
Café Del Mar, Vol. 11
Cirque Du Soleil Tapis Rouge
Desert Grooves 3
Deva Premal Embrace
Diane Arkenstone Aquaria: A Liquid Blue Trancescape
Erotic Lounge
Gabrielle Roth & The Mirrors Refuge

Gabrielle Rothe & The Mirrors Tongues
Le Groove Eclectique
Lovers Lounge
Moroccan Spirit
Songs of Kuan Yin
Tantra Lounge Vol. 3
Tantra Lounge Vol 4
Tantra Lounge Vol 5
Trance Yoga
Yoga Groove
Yoga Sol

You can find all of the music listed here on Amazon.com, where you can hear sample. All of the music is also linked from the Bondassage website.

The sound of your voice can also play into the sensuality of the scene. Although your partner will probably be wearing headphones while you are playing away, you may need to lift the headphones and give light commands ("Turn over so l can stroke you more"), or whisper sweet nothings into their ears from time to time so that they may get more aroused by your presence.

TASTE

Besides the obvious and often cliched references to the movie "9½ Weeks," the use of taste for erotic pleasure is largely overlooked. For your partner, under the complete control of your powerful charms, you can offer up some delectable tastes that harmonize perfectly with your orchestral maneuvers. Here are some sweet, sultry, clever, diabolical and plain ol' dirty ideas on how to play with taste.

Before the party begins, you may wish to start with an "aphrodisiac." Can certain foods really boost the libido? Possibly, but no matter what, if your taste buds are happy, and you believe in the power of the food to turn you on, then who's to say that a little ritual before play will do any harm? We say, indulge!

Here are a smattering of foods that are said to have abilities to increase your libido:

Chocolate
Chocolate has always been associated with love and romance—from the beginnings of the cacao in Aztec Civilization to today. What is it about chocolate and love that seem to go hand in hand? Well, chemicals! Chocolate contains theobromine and caffeine, (stimulants), phenylethylamine, (dopamine) and anandamide, (produces calm and well-being).

Oysters
These are better consumed before the massage than during! Oysters are high in zinc, which has been associated with improving sexual potency in men. Also, like other shell fish, oysters have also been thought to resemble female labia. Recently, mussels, clams and oysters have been found to contain compounds that may be effective in releasing sex hormones such as testosterone and estrogen.

Bananas
Bananas are phallic, and they are also high in potassium and B vitamins, which are said to be necessary for sex-hormone production. The reportedly arousing effects of

cucumbers, carrots, figs and avocados are also related to their looks.

Honey

Long associated with sex and fertility. Barbara Carellas, author of Urban Tantra, writes, "In medieval times, newlyweds would drink mead, a powerfully intoxicating fermented beverage made of honey and water, during the first month of marriage to increase virility and fertility. Thus, the first month of marriage became a honey-moon."

Offering tastes of food can be highly erotic for most people. Little nibbles between sexy talk or sensual touch can increase arousal immensely. You can also tease your partner by rubbing and drizzling tastes onto their body then licking them off either as the main event or between little tastes. Please be aware that sugary stuff in or near the vagina can increase the chance of infection. Best to keep honey on the breasts, back, knees, feet, etc.

Speaking of bodies, why not feed your partner a taste of your mouth, nipple, belly, vulva or penis in the same mindful, slow, teasing way you offered them a bite of fruit or chocolate? Take the time to savor each delicious morsel. And as the receiver, allow yourself to be tasted like the exotic delicacy you are.

Please be aware that in Bondassage we like using a bit of restraint, so don't put your partner in any danger of choking. If you are offering something large or chewy for them to taste, you may wish to sit them up first or start before they are restrained. For a lengthier, more atmospheric play, take the time to nibble, suck and drink from your earthly delights before tying them up. It will make the massage all the more erotic. Save some of the easier to consume tidbits like whipped cream or chocolate to nibble on during your play. Some fun ways of providing liquid while lying down is through a sippy cup, water bottles with flip tops and of course bendable straws.

Go slowly and enjoy the tastes of the world and each other!

BREATH AND SCENT

Breath is everything in life. It is the first thing we do when we enter the world and the last thing we do before we leave the world. Energy travels through breath and sexual energy is no exception. The more we breathe during sexual activity, the deeper we can go with our partner and the more aroused and alive we feel. Take a moment right now to breathe. Sit upright or lie down and start by taking a deep breath through your nose and into your belly. Let the air fill your belly as you breathe in pushing outward, like a Buddha belly and dropping your jaw, breathe out through your mouth, allowing all of that air to push outward as your belly contracts towards your spine. Repeat this process, perhaps counting to 4 or 6 as you breathe in and 6 or 8 as you breathe out. Notice what happens to your body and mind when you breathe deeply and consciously.

Breathing deeply through your nose like that will definitely open up your olfactory system, allowing you to really take in all the scents around you. We are a little fussy about smells in the U.S. Bombarded by deodorant, laundry and body soap, douching commercials subliminally telling us our bodies don't smell good, we seem to have lost touch of what sensual pleasures can arise from Mother Nature herself. What a shame.

Here are a few things you need to know about breath and sex:

Changing the way you breathe changes the way you feel.

Energy travels in the breath. Sexual energy is no exception. The deeper you breathe, the more you relax and become aware.

Intentional use of scent has always had the magical effect of unplugging our conscious mind and connecting us with our unconscious memories. It can lay the psychic and physical groundwork for intense arousal. Our sense of smell is directly linked to our sexuality in physical ways. The nose is lined with an erectile tissue similar to that of our nipples and genitals. When we smell scents that please us, the genital center is awakened. Perhaps you know of Marcel Proust's *Remembrance of Things Past* with his cup of tea and the madeleines? It's the smell that arouses him first, then the taste.

Like Proust, I'm sure you've had the experience of smelling something that immediately took you back to another time and place. You probably even experienced some of the same emotions you had felt at that time. Olfactory conditioning can be powerful, but it can also be quite subtle. For example, you might find yourself unexpectedly turned off by someone you had previously found magnetic if he were to wear the same cologne as an ex with whom you had a harsh break up.

Certain scents are historically believed to elicit sexual response. If you don't like any of these scents, obviously they will not be arousing for you. But if you aren't familiar with some of these, give them a try:

Musk - *Sexy And Sultry.*
Sandalwood - *Woody, Sensual.*
Patchouli - *Queen Of Sensuality! Potent.*
Ylang-Ylang - *Soothing, Relaxing.*

Rose - *Floral, Heady.*
Jasmine - *Deeply Hypnotic.*
Bergamot - *Perky, Sensual.*
Frankincense - *Warm, Inviting.*
Vanilla - *Sweet, Seductive.*
Neroli - *Sensual, Brightening.*

Start lightly and use the highest quality essential oils you can afford. A few high quality oils that assist your needs in the moment are better than overdoing it. Use scent in a variety of ways:

> *Try putting a couple drops on your fingertips, lightly tapping the forehead and temples of your partner.*
> *Burn it as incense in an oil infuser.*
> *Put a drop on top of an incandescent light bulb or on a candle.*
> *Add a few drops to a spray bottle of water for misting.*
> *Make your own aromatic combinations (vanilla and patchouli is wickedly sexy).*

If you want to further arouse your partner, you can also play with sensual erotic pulse points. There are six total and they can be found:

> *Between the little piece of cartilage at the front of the ear opening and the jaw.*
> *At the front of the neck between the voice box and adjacent muscle.*
> *Behind the clavicle, or collarbone. This may be a little tricky to find. Reach down inside the top edge of your collarbone and press down to feel the pulse.*

At the traditional pulse-taking point, located on the
thumb side of the wrist.
On the inside of the arm, at the elbow and below the bi-
ceps on the little-finger side of the tendon that runs down
the center of the arm.
Behind the knee.

The perspiration points are other scent amplification spots on
the body: between the breasts, the groin and under the arms.

Scent can be subtle, strong, complex or simple. Think about
how you wish to be thought of before application. Sweet and
floral scents recall a youthful femininity, spicy can connote passion, woody earthy and sensual, and citrus fresh and brightening. Imagine what you want to embody and signify that to your
lover through scent!

BONDAGE BASICS

"Surrender is a gateway to serenity and a portal to the pleasure you've been seeking."—Mistress C.

The success of any scene or exploration of BDSM is intimately linked to how well you know what you want and how clearly you ask for it. If you know what you want, you're more likely to receive it, especially when you make it your responsibility to find out what excites you and ask for it, or conversely, what excites your partner and provide it.

Mind reading is not a talent many people have. You can safely assume your partner is unable to read your mind to know what you want. Furthermore, *you* may not even know what you want, what you'd enjoy exploring or experiencing (or how, or where, or when...).

Before jumping into any new sensual or sexual exploration with your partner, we gently encourage you to take the time to determine what excites you. Good communication goes hand in hand with good sex. And good scenes leading to healthy and happy sensual explorations are best when built on a foundation of clear communication between partners.

Do yourself a favor and reflect solo or with your partner before your bedroom romp about what you would most enjoy. The clearer you are about this, the clearer your communication will be, and the more amazing your Bondassage or other sensual explorations will be, too.

Some questions to consider for opening the lines of communication and clarity:

> *What would be fun to me?*
> *What acts or implements have I never tried before that I've found myself curious about or drawn to?*
> *What have I experienced sensually or sexually in the past that I really enjoyed and would like to enjoy again?*
> *What have I seen other people do that I thought looked fun?*

Whether you're a true novice, an avid explorer, or a seasoned life-styler, when you know what you desire and what to ask for, you'll have much more fun. Remember, even if you are a seasoned player, today/right now is different from yesterday, tomorrow, or even two hours from now. Respect your different feelings and your partner's too. You'll be a more compassionate and caring partner. May you enjoy innumerable occasions of erotic excitement, abundance and well-being!

The easiest way to get started with bondage is with a set of restraint cuffs. They're simple to take on and off by buckling around the wrists or ankles. Adjustable to fit almost anyone, they won't tighten no matter how much the restrained partner pulls against them. This makes restraints a better choice than scarves, neckties or handcuffs: even fleece-lined toy handcuffs can cause damage to tendons and blood vessels. Make sure you can slip two fingers between the restraints and the wrists or ankles, since buckling them too tight could cut off blood flow to the hands and feet.

Different desires mean different approaches to bondage. For example, if your partner's fantasy is simply to relinquish control, choose lighter fabric restraints. Sportsheets makes great light-weight, sturdy, neoprene ones. If they want to pull and struggle, you'll need heavier leather restraints. It takes some time to learn the skills, but rope bondage can be as beautiful as it is func-tional. You may also wish to start by simply taking your part-ners hands and feet and put them where you want them, and tell them they are now tied in that position. This is a great non-threatening way to begin experimenting with bondage games should you and your partner feel so inclined.

Try tying your partner to the bed with their hands above their head, or try tying their feet to the legs of a chair. Adding a blind-fold will heighten their other senses, anticipating your every move. Tickle them with a feather or drip warm massage oil onto their skin. Almost any kind of sex play or sex toy can be incor-porated into bondage.

The more restrictive the bondage, the shorter the time some-one can stay bound. You have less time to play with someone tied standing up versus lying down. If you give your partner some wiggle room, you may be able to extend your play.

Surprises and emergencies happen, so be prepared to remove bondage quickly if necessary. Safety scissors can cut through rope without injuring skin: we recommend these for all rope play. Carabiners unclip in an instant and can also be used to at-tach rope to furniture. You can pick up safety scissors from any pharmacy and carabiners from most sports stores or hardware stores. Of course, you can probably get both online.

PADDLES AND FLOGGERS AND CROPS—OH MY!

"I adore playing my lover's body like a finely-tuned instrument"—June

In essence, Bondassage requires some sensory deprivation, light restraint and sensory play on your partner. We've discussed fun and sexy things like nipple clamps and fur mitts, but some people also appreciate a little more intensity. From a light, easy, fun spanking to things that may leave marks on your skin, we want to insure you know what you're doing and that you're doing it well. The following will help you to learn how to use your hand as a corporal tool and how to decide which tools to play with in scene. Although these tools can seem scary, you may also use them gently and lovingly, so remember, go slow and have fun!

Sting or Thud?

There is a general preference among people between the sensation of stingy or thuddy applications and implements. Let's determine the difference and how you may distinguish it for your partner, even if they don't know their preference.

Sting

A superficial pain that bites or tingles is called a sting. These sensations are generally harder for the receiver to process into desired pleasure than penetrating or thudding blows. Stingy strokes tend to make a sharp red mark. These are generally blows to a smaller surface area of the skin. Some implements that sting are: anything of a singular tube-like nature: switches, canes, plexi-rods, etc. Also rubber, plastic and metal sting more than leather (except the classic leather belt or more specialized whips like single tails), suede or fur. Finally, spanking tends to be more stingy than thuddy, but is a great way to stimulate your partner without tools and also creates a great "warm up" (getting their body prepared for further stimulation) for more intensity.

Thud

Blows fall over a broader area and tend to feel like massage stimulation. Thuddy implements tend to be made from denser materials and tend to leave a reddened area. Some common thuddy materials:

Heavy whips/floggers: these must have many wide tails —more than 9, usually made of heavy and/or soft leather like cow, elk, buffalo, or lamb. Fur floggers can be very sensual, and when made with sand stuffed into the fur tails, can be soft and thuddy simultaneously.

Most paddles are thuddy, although the thinner and lighter the paddle the more it will sting. People either tend to love or hate paddles, so take it slowly.

Some Things to Consider Beforehand

Bruising
Some people like having a few "marks" on their skin after play. It can be a great symbol of the intimacy shared. Usually light red marks will go away after a day or two, but sometimes the skin will bruise later. If you see bruising coming up during play, you will have bruising later. If there is any concern about bruising, go slowly, and if you see pink or redness, take a moment to caress the skin, then move from something heavier, such as a paddle, to something lighter, such as your hand. Some other considerations: avoid aspirin and anti-inflammatory drugs on the day you play. Ice afterwards.

Homeopathic Remedies
Arnica Montana ointment and tablets are a great healer for bruises. Traumeel ointment is a homeopathic ointment which is anti-inflammatory and an analgesic.

Some reasons for engaging in corporal play:

Reward vs. Punishment
We believe that corporal by and large is for reward, even if you're faking it as "punishment."

Heightening Intensity
Increased stimulation will increase intensity of your play.

Foreplay
Increasing intensity can lead to hotter sex!

Head Trip
A little bit of fear can make for a heady moment.

Ecstatic Journey
Guiding your partner on a sensual journey will always lead to more intimacy.

Role Play
Spanking from Aunty? Teacher disciplining a student? Role Plays can be lots of fun!

To Exert Control or Authority
Who's the boss?

Erotic Coercion
If you want (x, y or z), then you will need to take a whipping from me first...

Embarrassment
It can be a turn on for your partner to let them get spanked or paddled, naked and vulnerable, so be aware of this, even if they don't discuss it with you.

Emotional Release

Some people reach catharsis through tears, laughter or both while receiving corporal. Be sure to be patient and compassionate with yourself and your partner; and remember, you may not need to stop, just be fully present for them and check in.

Positions

Classic Bondassage is done on a massage table, to keep your partner in a comfortable position for an extended period of time while taking them on that exquisite journey.

But some people like to incorporate other options, and you may too, especially once you've mastered the basics. Consider your body position and body mechanics as well as your partner's. Make adjustments as necessary and change positions frequently. Never compromise safety.

Standing
On a cross or a post
On hands and knees
Kneeling
Laying down
Across the lap.
Over a chair or a desk
Spanking bench

Bear in mind space restrictions. For flogging, the optimal space is approximately 8 feet wide by 6-7 feet deep. Be aware of your surroundings—notice objects or people in the path of the whip.

Implements

Hands

Amazingly effective. While you are massaging your partner, you may give little slaps on the buttocks, creating more stimulation as you massage. Try light slapping all over the body, then try repetitive slapping on the buttocks to the rhythm of the music. It will be fun and heavenly for you both!

Paddles

Although they do not require a lot of training to use, paddles will bruise easily. Materials used in construction can include leather, rubber, wood, metal, composite materials, and common forms include leather strips, slappers, straps, frat paddles, ping pong or paddle ball paddles. Go lightly and if just starting out, don't forget to test it on the inside of your forearm and remember to warm up your partner.

Canes

Used ultra-lightly in a rhythmic fashion to the beat of the music, canes can be very stimulating, although for anything more aggressive, one needs to be properly trained in their use, as canes can be intense. There are two sensations with the cane, the initial sting and a few seconds later, the fire! Just remember, canes tend to mark, even when used lightly, so use with care. Canes are generally made from rattan. Bamboo tends to split, so it's not a good choice. Synthetic canes like fiberglass can leave marks that tend to stick around, so these are not a good choice for beginners.

Crops/Riding Crops

Crops are composed of a stiff shaft originally made from hickory (a dense, but flexible, switch wood), but usually now made from fiberglass or similar synthetic material, with a flap on the tip made of leather. These are fun and fairly easy to use. The leather flap makes a nice spot specific device.

Whips/Floggers/Cat o' Nine Tails

Made from leather, exotic hides, cotton, nylon, these are implements with a handle and one tail or multiple tails, which may be flat or braided. Some whips are easier to use, while others require instruction and lots of practice (eg, the singletail and bullwhip). Be mindful of the "wrap" effect: allowing the tips of a whip or cane to curl around to strike parts of the body other than the intended target. For example, aiming for the behind, but letting the tips of the whip wrap around and strike the hip bone. Bruising on the hips is often a sign of a careless or incompetent flogger who is frequently unaware of the damage that is occurring. To get started with Bondassage, we suggest a light, fluffy, short tailed, soft leather flogger, using it to "brush" the skin.

Belts

Soft, thick leather is ideal. Fold the belt over in half and hold just the other side of the buckle. Of course, be careful of buckles and studs.

Flogger and Whip Safety

Try not to break the skin!

Leather cleaners and conditioners will not be able to guarantee cleanliness—so don't let bodily fluids come into direct contact with your leather toys.

For using on pussy/cock/balls, use one made of plastic, rubber or PVC that can be washed and cleaned effectively, or dedicate a leather toy for use with just one person.

Where to Spank, Flog, etc.

If you're new to corporal, start by focusing your attention on the buttocks. Butt cheeks are usually pretty well-padded and less prone to injury. Draw a heart shape around the butt with your finger tips: this is the erotic zone. The underside of the bottom is called the "sweet meat" because the nerves that run from there go straight to the genitals. When struck just so, they send little messages of eroticization.

In general, safe places to strike are the places with a fair amount of fat or with a lot of muscle. The most popular areas for striking are the buttocks and the muscled parts of the upper and middle back. Thighs are OK, but be careful about the sides of the hips, which tend to be very sensitive on most people. There are lots of important nerves that run through these areas and the bones are rather close to the surface.

Be careful, too, about the insides of the thighs. Although this area is safe to hit, it is also very sensitive, and the pain potential is quite high here.

The upper back on either side of the spine is protected by a thick layer of muscle. The shoulder blades are relatively close to the surface. You can flog these areas with soft, flexible whips of leather and perhaps even rubber, but you will want to avoid using paddles, canes and the shafts of crops so that you don't bruise the bones. A lot of people really enjoy being beaten on their upper backs since it can feel like a vigorous massage and is a logical continuation of the massage you are giving.

Of course you want to be careful to avoid hitting the tailbone, and never strike strongly any soft organs such as the kidneys.

Warming Up

All recipients need a warm up before increasing intensity. Even if you are playing punishment games, you will need to warm them up, perhaps with a stricter demeanor to make up for it. In Bondassage, your receiver is usually already relaxed from the massage, on a delicious musical journey, and ready for a bit more intensity. Starting lightly with hands slapping across the body, soft floggers whipped lightly up and down the body, or light canes tapped or bounced on the fleshy parts gently. The "warm up" may be sufficient for some. Better to keep it light and find out they wanted more, than to overdo it!

Corporal Play

Spanking

Hands are your best friends when it comes to spanking. As mentioned above, while massaging your partner try some light slapping, then try variety like spreading your fingers or keeping your palm flat, you'll get more sting. If you bring your fingers together or cup your hand, you'll get more thud and you can caress the bottom between strokes!

Implements

Although some people prefer a hands-on approach, toys provide sensations of their own. After your own skin, leather slappers are the next-best choice. Paddles can be constructed from almost any material: the more rigid they are, the stronger the sensation. Strike with the middle of the paddle, not the edge. Canes and crops can be used for a quick stinging slap or swung whistling through the air to create incredibly strong sensations.

Soles of the Feet

Some people like the bottoms of their feet beaten and others do not! There are a lot of bones close to the surface of the feet, so whatever you decide to do, be cautious. Tickling may be more appropriate.

Genitals

These are very sensitive areas which can be whipped with great care. Use only very soft whips made of deerskin or lambskin at first—and dedicate the use of that implement to that person alone if you will be contacting bodily fluids. Experiment carefully with heavier toys later. Besides the obvious clustering of nerves on and around the vulva, there are sensitive glands that can become irritated. Some cock and balls like intense treatment, but most do not. As always, start lightly to gauge how your partner responds. Some women enjoy spanking or whipping of their vulva, but the area can become desensitized with a lot of intense stimulation. Discuss your partner's preference for this and proceed wisely.

Breasts

Breasts are mostly comprised of fat. There are quite a few nerves at the nipples and surrounding the aureole. Women differ greatly in sensitivity and enjoyment in having their

breasts stroked intensely. As with the genitals, start lightly
and proceed as necessary for the scene.

The Forearms
Forearms are relatively free of dangerous areas, but they
are also relatively free of erotic areas. There are many deli-
cate bones in the wrists, and they are very nice to lovingly
stroke and nibble upon. The palms of the hands are an-
other one of those like it/hate it areas.

Face Slapping
This can be done with care. Give light, open-handed slaps
to the cheeks, using your finger pads. Hold the face with
the opposite hand to keep it stabilized. Light taps can be
stimulating in an "embarrassing" turn on way. Of course,
some people cannot tolerate face slapping. Be sure to ne-
gotiate this ahead of time.

Now that you have more knowledge on corporal and its myri-
ad implements, you are ready to make that sensual connection
with your partner.

Remember, if new to an implement, test it on the inside of
your forearm. You may also wish to set aside "practice" time
with your partner, asking for feedback as you go along, so that
when you are actually playing you will feel more confident and
less in need of constant check-ins. Of course, reading your partner's body language and ideally moans and groans will also in-
form you of how much deeper you can go together.

Finally, don't forget you are striking a person, not a "thing"...
always stay connected through breathing, coming from your
heart and through your hands. Enjoy!

*"I love the meditative quality of Bondassage
and all that it has to offer."—Eve*

TICKLES & PRICKLES & SIGHS

"The ultimate sensual gift, for you and your partner!"—Doug and Jennifer

Some things tickle, some things prickle, and all things can potentially bring a sigh of pleasure. Once you've created a lovely sensual atmosphere, talked about safety, negotiated what you're each comfortable with, and acclimated yourself with your tools, then you can start to play with some of the sensations these tools bring, using your skills and imagination! The things you do may prick and tickle, but the goal is always to induce sighs of pleasure.

SENSATION PLAY IDEAS

As we've already stated, there's a lot to be said for the sensations your body receives once blindfolded. The following are some ideas on what to play with and then how to utilize some of them in scene to keep the flow...

Heat

Wax (candle, paraffin, not beeswax—it gets too hot!)
Hot Water (use an eyedropper)
Hot Breath
Warm Washcloth
The Following are for external use only:
  Cayenne Pepper
  Ginger
  Capsicum
  Cinnamon Oil
  Wasabi
  Tiger Balm
Hand Warmers For Skiing

Cold

Ice
Ice Cups (freeze water in small Dixie cups)
Ice Cubes
Once again, external use only:
  Polar Lotion/Icy Hot
  Canned Air Spray
  Menthol
  Listerine or other mouth strips
  Altoids
Pearls
Chain
Knife (blunt side only please!)

Soft

Fur, real or fake (mitts, bits from coats: rabbit, mink)
Feathers

Satin
Silk Scarf
Paint Brushes
Makeup Brush
Silicone Basting Brushes
Artist's Brushes
Cotton Swab
Flogger
Long Hair
Cornstarch (drop in "plops" on the skin)

Scratchy

Vampire Gloves (leather gloves covered in tiny spikes, available from fetish shops and sex toy retailers—be careful about drawing blood unless for single person use)
Wartenberg Wheel
Wool
Forks
Bottle caps
Metal Hair Brushes
Whisks
Toothpicks
Combs
Fingernails
Gravel
Brush (bath brushes, hair brushes, paint brushes)
Pipe cleaners
Loofah
Sponges
Dishwashing Pad
Bath Gloves

Sandpaper
Emery Board
Tingler (copper head massager)

Smooth

Leather
Suede
Chamois
Rubber Sheeting
Neoprene
Liquid Latex
Glass (you can find glass toys made for body use)
Pyrex
Plastic
Metal, especially stainless steel
Smooth Wood
Wax Paper

Pinchy

Clothespins
Clips
Clamps
Biting
Pinching
Plastic Vise Grips
Alligator Clips
Pickle Tongs
Practice Drumsticks (good for rhythmic body percussion)

Suction

Snakebite Kit

Sucking
Cupping Sets (made for sensual use or acupuncture)

Vibration
Disposable Electric Toothbrushes
Vibrators:
  Bullets
  Rabbit
  Hitachi Magic Wand: with attachments

Percussion
Canes
Paddles
Hands—fists, open palms
Flogging
Rubber Bands (stingy)
Studded Paddle
Crops
Wooden Spoons
Practice or Regular drumsticks

Smell
Essential Oils
Flowers
Pine Branches
Citrus (brightening)
Vanilla (sensual)
Cinnamon (exotic awakening)
Basil (clearing)
Patchouli (sensual)

Taste

Needless to say, external use only:
Popsicles
Chocolate
Honey
Jam
Whipped Cream
Breath Mints
Flavored Lip Gloss

Heat and Cold (menthol/capsicum) are not designed, intended or recommended for internal use (except for the foods, which are intended for use in the mouth only.) We do not recommend using them inside the genitals or anus. These substances can also upset the natural biological balance of such areas.

A very small amount of a cream or lubricant sold as a "hot sex" substance can, in some cases, be applied to genitals to make masturbation more intense, but please be careful. Remember, these substances are not intended for internal use, and it feels much "hotter" on mucous membranes. For women, we suggest you try this on your own before involving another person. Menthol-containing cough drops might be used during cunnilingus, but please note the above warnings carefully. These substances must be used cautiously. Start slowly and with small amounts when using a commercially produced "hot sex" cream or lubricant. It's often wise to dilute it with another lubricant, at least at first. If it is oil-based, combine it with an oil based lube, if it is water-based, combine with a water-based lube. Never use the extra-strength brand of anything until you've used the regular strength brand successfully several times. Understand that gels can be much hotter than creams.

"Hot sex" substances may take up to 5 minutes for the effects of a given "dose" to be fully felt, so take your time about adding more. One dose is usually felt for about 20 minutes, but this can vary considerably from person to person and from product to product. Such substances applied to the scrotum are usually felt sooner and feel hotter than the same substance applied to the penis. Be careful about combining these substances with abrasion. Skin that has been scraped, such as by fingernails, will be considerably less able to tolerate such play.

It's easy to add more of whatever substance you're using, but it's very difficult to remove what you've already applied. If you do have a "hot sex overdose," you can usually wash it off by using cold running water and lots of soap. Applying large amounts of shampoo and then washing it off works especially well. Liberal amounts of witch hazel can also cool things down, as can generous amounts of petroleum jelly or an oil-based cream.

Because most of these substances "burn" for about 20 mins after being applied (some brands burn longer), and because this feeling may be seriously unpleasant if no longer accompanied by sexual arousal, it's both wise and compassionate to wait for its sensations to fade to a very low level before bringing your partner to orgasm.

As you can see, "hot sex" is one of the more serious tricks, with a steeper learning curve than most. Starting lightly, like using cough drops or mints while performing oral, and if your partner enjoys that sensation perhaps moving onto a frugal application of menthol rub on the genitals, can add extraordinary sensations to your scene.

More Fun with Vibrators

Try using a vibrator on various parts of your genitals—many guys enjoy the vibration on their penis (particularly on the underside just below the head if circumcised), their perineum, (the place between the shaft of the penis and the anus), and their anus. If it's her vibrator you're using, or if you want to use it on someone else later, cover it carefully with a condom, rubber glove, or plastic wrap, or put plastic wrap over the part of you that you're stimulating.

Hold a vibrator against the base of his cock while performing fellatio. Take his penis into your mouth, then apply a vibrator to your cheek. Move the vibrator sensuously from one cheek to the other. Touch it to your lips. Apply it to the point of your chin. Turn your head so that the head of his penis makes a bulge in one of your cheeks and apply the vibrator to that bulge.

Attach a small, battery-operated vibrator to the underside of your tongue during oral sex, thus turning your tongue into a vibrating sex toy.

Take a sip of champagne or sparkling water, hold it in your mouth, and insert his penis, (this can be very intense). Now touch a vibrator to your cheek and notice his reaction.

Put an ice cube (one with no sharp edges or corners) in your hand, and apply your hand to his well-lubricated penis. Now touch a vibrator to the base of his penis while you masturbate him.

Encircle the top of his scrotum with your thumb and forefinger. Squeeze this ring together until it's snug and his testicles are "trapped" below it, then slowly pull down until the skin of his scrotum is pulled tight over his testicles. Now apply your vibrator to the tight-skinned sack.

Many men find wonderful surprises when a vibrator hums up

against the frenulum, which is the inverted "V" area on the underneath side of the head of the penis. This is a "must try" for men who insist vibrators have no erotic effect on them.

Another exciting area for many women and men is from immediately behind the genitals to near the bottom of the spine. Many nerve endings here come alive during sexual arousal. As you slide your vibrator along this area, be careful not to move microorganisms from the anus to the vagina or to the penis. Another option is to vibrate through a small towel that remains stationary on the pelvic floor. Also, be cautious with vibrators on scrotums. With some types of vibrators, it might be very painful.

In your own erotic investigations, you may have found other exciting places. Play with them too. And don't forget between the toes.

Good Vibrations Hug

Fully clothed and standing up, invite your lover to share a hug. Nestle your turned-on vibrator into a comfortable position between your pubic areas. Then hug for five minutes. Don't let go. Don't fall down. And make certain there aren't any urgent appointments following this hug—you would probably be late.

Brush Off

A large soft brush can create a thrilling sensation. You can buy paint brushes from an art supply store, or makeup brushes or shaving brushes from the drugstore. The brush can be used for delightful teasing as well as to bring your partner to orgasm (use it without lube.) Hold her vaginal lips open with one hand and use the brush on the inside of her outer lips, on her inner lips (using both back and forth and up and down motions), and on her clit (top to bottom may work especially well).

Some women can orgasm by having a vibrator held firmly against the bottoms of their feet.

Try combining a vibrator with a vaginal speculum. Try inserting the speculum, opening it a bit and holding a vibrator against the base. If that gets a promising reaction, you can try opening it a bit more, then a bit more, so you're putting tension against the walls of the vagina. You may get a truly spectacular reaction.

Playing Chopsticks

Combine a long, narrow, rigid implement such as a chopstick with a strong vibrator to vibrate into tiny little places, or to sharply localize the vibration to a larger place. Hold the chopstick loosely in one hand with its tip against the part you want to stimulate, then touch the vibrator to its base.

Variant on Bath Mitts

Especially the ones with one smooth side and one textured side, are wonderful for slowly stimulating and soothing your partner's skin. Some mitts have a little "pocket" designed for slipping a bar of soap in while showering. Placing a few marbles in that pocket can create a wonderful sensation.

The above tips and tricks are obviously only the tip of the iceberg. Your imagination is your best friend when it comes to erotic play. Once you know how to use lubes, creams and sharp things safely, you will be able to enjoy all that you and your partner can imagine together.

SAMPLE SEQUENCES

"Bondassage provides a wonderfully unique opportunity to share deep pleasure with each other. We knew it would be good, but we had no idea how good."—Tom and Stan

Now that you've learned about negotiating with your partner, safety procedures, bondage techniques, implements and how to use them, and of course massage practices, you are ready to start putting your first Bondassage scene together.

Whether you are getting your feet wet in the practice or expanding your already spicy sex life, we want you to be able soar through your scene with confidence, sensuality, spice and love. You may wish to start small, maybe organizing a one hour scene or more and see where that takes you, or you may wish to dive into a deep three hour intensive scene—either way, you will increase the intimacy you and your partner share and become more fluent in the alternative languages of love.

The following scenarios are meant to serve as a recipe book. They can set you up for a perfect scene, or you may use them as springboards to begin your erotic journeying together:

THE TASTY TEASER
(30–60 MINUTES)

Ask your partner to lie face down on the bed or massage table. Instruct them to not move a muscle or you'll stop whatever wicked delight that you're doing. You may also lightly tie their wrists and ankles apart with soft rope or light restraints.

Put the blindfold and the headphones (or earbuds) on your partner and check for comfort. Choose one or two sensation play items, (like a furry mitt and electric toothbrush), and one percussion implement (like a paddle or leather strap), and don't forget your hands.

With bare hands or maybe corn starch, begin by lightly stroking and rocking your lover's body starting with the back and shoulders and working your way down and up again. If using corn starch, wipe it off sensually with a fluffy towel. Then, using warm oil for massage, alternate periods of sensual touch with periods of light sensation play. Tickle your partner on the bottom and groin areas, then use a fur mitt or light paddle to stimulate the area. Visit the genitals and the bottom often. Wipe off the oil or massage cream with hot towels and finish the face-down sequence with some nice, slow soft body percussion (flogging and spanking are lovely here).

Before beginning the body percussion, wipe your lover down with a hot wet towel and dry them off. You want to remove as much of the oil or massage cream as you can to keep your floggers and percussion instruments clean. Alternately, you could cover your lover with a satin sheet and do your percussion through that.

Ask your partner to turn over, adjusting the blindfold and headphones. Put their arms above their head or out to the sides of their body, ankles apart, and either tie them lightly or instruct them not to move a muscle.

Begin by using soft sensation play items (fur mitts, satin pillowcases, feathers), slowly up and down the body. Pour warm oil or massage cream into your hands and slowly and lovingly massage your partner, starting at the chest and working down the front of the body. Alternate periods of massage with periods of light sensation play. Again, if you'd like to use a flogger on them and don't want to get it greasy, simply cover the area with the satin pillowcase and flog them through that.

Vary the rhythm of your caresses and begin paying more attention to the genitals. Increase and decrease the amount of sexual energy you are building. Use a variety of strokes, pressures and tempos with your hands, vibrator or toys.

Remember, each person is different, so on one day you may want to use your hands and give "permission" to release, on another day, you may wish to "take" what you want. As the giver, you get to decide. As receiver, you will want to surrender to the giver's desire. This sequence is great for beginners, when you have less time, or when you are exploring new touch or a new partner.

THE DELIGHTFUL DINNER
(1–2 HOURS)

Have your partner disrobe and use the bathroom if necessary. Ask them to kneel down naked before you and place their hands behind their back. If you like, fasten a collar around their neck, checking to see that you can still slip two fingers underneath. Ask for their hands, one at a time, and fasten on wrist cuffs. Jaeleen likes to take her partner's hand and place it on the upper part of her breast. It provides a stable, tantalizing position to attach the cuffs.

Once you've attached cuffs to your lover's wrists, ask them to (gracefully) stand up and spread their legs. Many people are uncomfortable standing with their hands at their sides, so in Bondassage we like to give them something to do with their hands. Ask them to place them either behind their neck or on top of their head— this has the added benefit of being a lovely posture exercise. Kneel down and attach the cuffs to the ankles, taking the time to lovingly stroke and compliment them.

Face Down Sequence

Ask your lover to lay face down on the massage table or the bed. Place a pillow under their hips and spread their legs apart. If your partner has a penis, reach between the legs and pull it down so it points towards their feet. Put the blindfold and the headphones on, checking for comfort.

Tie wrists and ankles to the legs of the massage table or out to the sides of the bed. You can prepare the bed ahead of time by placing rope on headboard and footboard or you can run rope between the mattress and the box spring so that it is sticking out at each corner, ready to use.

Follow the same sequence as described in the previous sequence, "The Tasty Teaser," moving more slowly and deliberately. Lightly stroke the entire body using hands/fur mitts/satin pillowcase/feathers from the upper body to the feet. Apply warm lotion to the entire back of the body. Massaging slowly and lovingly, alternate periods of touch with periods of sensation play. Choose 3–5 different items—a vibrating toothbrush is one of our favorites. Make sure to gently visit the genitals and bottom often. For example, you might run a feather over the body, then massage the back, then massage the ass, then massage the legs, then tickle the genitals with the toothbrush, then massage the head, then spank a little with hands, then use a leather paddle for a bit, then rub a fur mitt on the recipient's warm ass.

Before beginning the body percussion, wipe your lover down with a hot wet towel and dry them off. You want to remove as much of the oil or massage cream as you can to keep your floggers and percussion instruments clean. Alternately, you could cover your lover with a satin sheet and do your percussion through that.

We like to start with some slow, sensual spanking, followed by flogging and (perhaps) cropping or caning. Choose 2 or 3 implements (or let your partner choose before you start). Begin by keeping your movements slow and soft and build the intensity, backing off every so often to spread the sensations throughout the body.

To continue to build sensuality, fondle and caress the genitals, insert a finger or a toy. Let the toy be your "other hand" and continue the massage, perhaps adding a vibrator, more fingers, toys etc. Use your imagination. Eve loves doing a full on "bodyslide": Naked, mount the table or bed and put a fair amount of oil on your chest (this works particularly well if the receiver is still tingling from spanking, paddling, or caning). Now gently move to the music into the backside of your partner, rubbing your body along theirs until your bodies completely converge. If you have an ample chest (like us!), then use your breasts as another massage tool. The bodyslide is guaranteed to make your lover shudder with delight!

Cool things back down by slowly running your hands over their skin. Finish with a minute or two of stillness. When you're ready, untie them, remove pillow from under hips and ask them to turn over.

Face Up Sequence

Check in with your lover to see how they're doing and to see if they need water, tissue, or a bathroom break (or if you prefer, just pay close attention. You should be able to see if they are blissed or needing). Place a pillow under their head, adjust the blindfold and headphones, and retie their limbs. Tie their legs apart (not too far if their hips are tight), and tie the arms overhead or at their sides (if at their sides, they may drop down unless you run your rope over and under the massage table. Don't worry, when you practice you'll see what works best for you.

Begin as you did with the Face Down Sequence. Lightly stroke down entire front of body with your hands, followed by stroking with fur, satin and feathers. Optional: Apply warm oil or lotion to the entire front of the body. Jaeleen likes to apply lotion to the legs and feet and skip the torso. This keeps the sensation play toys cleaner.

Massaging slowly and lovingly, alternate periods of touch with periods of sensation play. We call this "freeform" in Bondassage. Use your hands, mouth, fingernails, feathers, fur, vibrating toothbrushes, hair brush, tools, ice... mix it up. Keep it very slow, soft and sensual. Visit the genitals often to keep them aroused and revisit the chapter on erogenous zones section for ideas on building the energy.

You can finish the session in a variety of ways. If your partner is ready (and you're willing for them to) orgasm, you can:

Untie their hands and let them pleasure themselves. You can "assist" by using your hands or mouth, or by using a vibrator or toy on them.

Take them there yourself. Climb up between their legs, sit astride the table with their legs draped over yours, or stand off to one side and help them achieve an ecstatic release with your hands and/or vibrator.

Remove the headphones off and coach them through the Clench and Hold (as described in the Pussy Pleasure and Penis Pleasure chapters) to retain and spread the sexual energy you've built.

Slow the tempo down—either gradually or abruptly—and leave them "hot and bothered."

However you choose to end the session, we love to place warm wet towels on the genitals and chest, uncuff their wrists and ankles and tuck them snugly under a soft blanket. Let them float. Stay close by but don't touch them. Allow them to absorb and process the delicious journey you've taken them on.

When they come back to earth (you'll notice their breathing changing, or perhaps they wiggle their fingers and toes), slowly remove the headphones and blindfold. Stay silent—this is not the time for chit chat. If we get a "Wow—that was amazing" out of our partners, that's just lovely. Massage your lover's head, neck, shoulders. Praise them for being brave/responsive/hot/fun and snuggle them. End the session with a leisurely shower or bath, and a delicious treat.

THE BEAUTIFUL BUFFET
(3+ HOURS)

As Einstein said, "...Imagination is more important than knowledge. Knowledge is limited. Imagination encircles the world." If you have the luxury of an extended amount of time, the sky's the limit.

Bearing in mind all of the basics above, you may also choose to combine any of the following suggestions:

> *Extend the collaring and cuffing ritual. Eve has a wealth of information and brilliant techniques for this. Contact her directly for a skype or phone coaching session or check out your local Kink community for classes.*

> *Take turns—each of you receiving Bondassage for an hour or so, with a break for snacks and clean up in between. Flip a coin to see who receives first or negotiate using our suggestions.*

> *Focus entirely on one of you and try all the toys and goodies at your disposal. Conversely, you might just choose one sensation play item and one percussion implement. Dive deep and discover twenty things you never knew you could do with a hairbrush.*

> *Incorporate a "tasting menu"—feed your lover different delightful tidbits in addition to sensual touch, sensation play and body percussion.*

Slow yourself down. If you think you are going slowly, go slower. See if you can go half as slow as you normally do. Mix it up, try going super-slow, then fast. Alternate rhythm based on the music.

Work on the entire body except the genitals, then start again, integrating the genitals.

Talk dirty to your partner. Lift up the headphones and tell them they are your captive and you will use them however you like. Call them "toy" or "slut" with an appreciative voice. Encouraging them to moan and groan loudly. Start with a Tantric exercise before you begin. Barbara Carellas is our go to source for all things Tantra and beyond, and her book Urban Tantra *contains many examples complete with instructions. We like the Yab Yum and bathing rituals.*

Bring in a friend and see how much variety can occur when 4 hands are involved!

Once they are tied down and aroused, sit back and watch your partner. Tell them how beautiful, how vulnerable they are. Move back in slowly with caresses, strokes, and more caresses, continuing to admire specific body parts as you play with them.

Whatever you choose, be mindful of the energy. Just because "5 hours sounds fantastic" doesn't mean that it's a great idea. Shorter sessions can be better (especially as you're developing your skills and your connection) and it's always nicer to leave them wanting more. Conversely, if you are really enjoying yourselves and are not pressed for time, you may find yourselves playing for hours without realizing it. Insuring you have a delicious meal and a bit of down time available after will help you both ease back into the "real world."

AFTERCARE

*"After the decadence of your sensual massage
and sensation play, hot towels and a soft,
cozy blanket will further relax you. Lay
in this warm embrace."—Lorna*

Aftercare is the time you and your partner take afterwards to recuperate. For some people, that may mean a glass of water and a bit of a cuddle, others may wish to talk about the experience, some may need full on snuggles, cuddles, blankets and rest. In other words, aftercare varies widely from person to person and from situation to situation. What we do recommend is having fresh water and a blanket nearby as basic material needs. Your receptivity to whatever condition your partner is in without judgment and with compassion will be the most essential aspect to consider for after care. Ask if they would like water and the blanket, then ask if they wish to cuddle or be left alone. Most people will have some idea on the basics. If not, simply sit next to them until they are ready to reach out to you or speak.

AFTERCARE NOTES

Stay present

Don't talk or touch. Breathe together.

Gently fold the sheet around the body. They may want their face covered.

Just let them be for 15-30 minutes. Allow whatever happens to happen.

When they're ready to move

Help them roll onto their side and eventually, to sit up.

Provide water, food, chocolate, warmth, blanket, cuddling, nap, sleep, sex, more sex?

Our genitals remain very sensitive after we've had sex. One thing that can feel wonderful is to moisten a washcloth with warm water and place it there. Safety note: Make sure the water is comfortably warm, but not too hot. Test it on the inside of your elbow before placing it on them.

After sex, many people like to cuddle, but they may also be hungry or thirsty too. After a few minutes of cuddling, a considerate partner might discreetly disengage himself and go fetch something to drink and eat. Having these stashed close to the bedroom lessens the time you are away from your partner and sends the message that you care enough to plan ahead.

Check in

Whether you live with your partner or not, be sure to send a little note of consideration a couple days later checking in to see how they feel. Some people need a bit of time to process the sensations they've received. Remember to keep an open mind and heart to what they tell you. Being told you are wonderful is wonderful, but hearing about what doesn't work for them is just as essential, that way you can create a more intensely beautiful experience each and every time.

You don't have to do this right away, but it's a good idea to spend some time after your session talking about what went well, and what didn't. If something you do in your session really turned your partner off, try not to take it personally. You wouldn't be human if you didn't take it somewhat personally, but try not to buy into that too deeply. Remember, each person has their own pattern of desires and turn-offs, and you can never completely know what that pattern looks like.

"My whole body is smiling."—Teddy

FINAL NOTES

We live in a society that portrays sex as if we all magically know how to do it with each other without talking about it, which is simply not true. Take it from your friendly "sexperts" here that practice, conversation, moving slowly, more conversation, empathy and compassion will all make for more connection and deeper intimacy. You may eventually appear as though you're reading your partner's mind, but like any good improv person knows, you make it look easy through practice. Further, even if you are tying your lover up and doing "wicked" things to them, which may look scary to the untrained eye, if you follow your heart and remain connected, you will always deepen your practice, becoming a better lover and a better partner.

Bondassage came about from many years of experience, and we've condensed it down to simple, easy-to-use practices. Through trial and error, we have learned a lot, and we want you to have the best possible experience you can. We hope you've found our little book to be helpful in your life and love.

In Kink and Love,
Jaeleen and Eve
August, 2013

GLOSSARY

Some of the terms listed here occur in the text, while we have included some others you may have heard bandied about in relation to BDSM play and other forms of power exchange. To learn more, please visit our extensive resources page on the Bondassage website.

Aftercare *A time after a sex or play session in which to calm down, cuddle and slowly come back in touch with reality.*

Anal Play *Sexual activity such as rimming, anal intercourse, and play with insertable toys.*

Bathtub Fantasies *Fantasies that fall into the realm of "really hot to think about but best left in the mind."*

BDSM *Bondage and Discipline, Dominance and Submission, Sadism and Masochism. A combined acronym often used as a catchall for anything in the kink scene.*

Bear's Paw *Fur gloves used for sensation play which have blunt metal spikes or dull hooks at the end of each fingertip.*

Bondage *Securing someone physically with restraints— rope, chains, cuffs, rubber, plastic wrap. Bondage typically refers to total restraint, however it can be limited to a particular body part, such as breast bondage.*

Bottom *In BDSM lingo, the recipient of activities—the one "done-to" rather than the "do-er." The receptive person in a relationship or play setting.*

Boundaries *Established limits (soft or hard) as to what you will or will not do.*

Butt Plug *A sex toy intended for anal stimulation, consisting of a flared dildo, usually quite short, with a wide base, designed to remain securely in the anus until removed. They come in a variety of sizes; some vibrate.*

Cane *A thin, flexible instrument used to strike a person. Canes are often made of rattan or a similar material, but may be made of other types of wood or even of flexible plastic such as polycarbonate. They are quite painful, often leaving marked welts. Also means to strike with a cane, "to cane."*

Cat o' Nine Tails *A multi-tailed whip with weighted or knotted ends.*

Clover Clamp *A specific type of nipple clamp consisting of a clamp with a lever mechanism to which a chain or cord is affixed in such a way that pulling on the chain or cord increases pressure on the clamp.*

Cock Ring *A ring (often made of metal or rubber) or strap designed to be affixed around the base of an erect penis. The ring allows blood to flow into the penis but constricts the penis sufficiently to prevent blood from flowing out, preventing the penis from becoming flaccid once it is erect.*

Collar *An item worn around the neck, frequently leather or chain, sometimes equipped with a locking device to prevent its removal. Often worn as a symbol of submission.*

Condition (v) *To develop a reflex or behavior pattern or to cause to become accustomed to. Much of D/s slave training relies on these techniques.*

Consent *Approval or permission freely given in a context for someone to engage in a particular activity without coercion. Informed consent is consent freely given beforehand and being fully aware of the conditions and consequences of the activity.*

Corporal Punishment *Punishment inflicted directly on the body, such as whipping, caning, or spanking.*

Crop *A thin, flexible instrument used for striking, consisting of a rigid but flexible shaft wrapped with leather or a similar material, with a handle at one end and often* with a small leather loop at the other. Also means to strike with a crop.

D/s *The shorthand term for Dominance/Submission.*

Discipline *Punishment or correction; or the training of a submissive.*

Dom/Domme *Man or woman who takes control or authority, ruling, prevailing, the one who prefers to be on "top." The words Dom and Domme are pronounced the same way—Domme refers to a female authority. Also known as Domina or Dominatrix. Some find use of the terms Dom /Domme and Sub gives their Bondassage play an extra charge.*

Dominant *Someone who has a desire to control or have power over another and/or assumes the dominant role in sex or playtime.*

Edge Play *SM play that involves a chance of harm, either physically, emotionally, or psychologically. Because the definition of edge play is subjective to the specific players (i.e., what is risky for me may not be as risky for you), there isn't a universal list of what is included in edge play. However, there are a few forms of play which almost always make the cut; including fire play, gun play, rough body play, breath play and blood play.*

E-stim *The use of made-for-erotic-use electrical stimuli to create a desired sensation.*

Endorphins *Naturally-occurring opiate-like chemicals produced in the brain in response to pain, which block pain and can produce a euphoric sensation. The euphoria sometimes described by people who engage in BDSM is often attributed to endorphins.*

Exhibitionism *The act of publicly exposing parts of one's body that are conventionally covered, especially in seeking sexual gratification or stimulation.*

Fetish *Any thing or activity to which one is irrationally devoted; any object, sexual or nonsexual, which excites erotic feelings.*

Fire & Ice *The use of hot (as in wax) and cold (as in ice) for sexual stimulation.*

Fisting *The practice of inserting the entire hand into the vagina or into the anus. Fisting is actually quite a bit easier to do than most people realize; the human body is quite accommodating. The fingers are placed together and inserted slowly; as the hand is inserted, the fingers tend to curl into a loose ball. Many people experience intense orgasms from fisting.*

Flogger *Any multi-lashed whip typically made of leather, but may also be made of materials such as rope, suede, horsehair, or other types of hide.*

Flying, or Floating *Rare and special transcendent state of consciousness achieved during a scene.*

Foot Fetish *Sexual obsession for the feet or shoes.*

Gag *Device placed in the mouth to stop or stifle vocal sounds.*

Going Under *Term describing a receiver or bottom's emotional state when totally immersed in a fantasy.*

Golden Shower *Urination on another person.*

Hard Limit *What someone absolutely will not do—not negotiable.*

Head Games *Domination where the focus is mostly mental, as in humiliation play.*

Humiliation or Embarrassment Play *Playful humbling or teasing of a person that creates arousal.*

Impact Play *Any activity involving striking or hitting. For example: spanking, flogging, or caning.*

Insertables *Anything (dildos, butt plugs) inserted into a bodily opening—i.e. the ass, pussy or mouth—for sexual purposes. These should be covered with a condom before play for safety and easy clean up.*

Latex *Rubber material used in making tight, or restrictive, fetish clothing; often a fetish object in itself.*

Lifestyle *Referring to involvement in BDSM (i.e. "How long have you been in the lifestyle?"). Sometimes also referred to as "the scene."*

Limits *Boundaries the dominant and submissive set for each other during the talk-it-over stage regarding do's and don'ts during the scene.*

Masochism *The act of receiving pain, (extreme sensation), for sensual or sexual pleasure.*

Masochist *One who gets pleasure from physical or psychological pain, either inflicted by others or self-inflicted.*

Master or Mistress *Someone who identifies with a lifestyle choice to dominate someone (a slave)—sometimes 24/7.*

Mental Bondage *Assuming a bondage position on command and "holding it" as if tied in ropes.*

Milking *Stimulating a man's prostate with a dildo or finger to produce an ejaculation without orgasm.*

Over-the-Knee (OTK) *Classic spanking position.*

Paddle *A rigid, flat implement made of wood or leather used to smack a bottom.*

Pain Slut *Slang for a masochist who derives pleasure from physical pain.*

Pervertable *Everyday household objects, like clothespins for nipple clamps or paint stirrers for paddles, that can be "converted or perverted" for kinky play.*

Percussion Play *Using an instrument designed to strike with force, typically a flogger, paddle or cane.*

Position Training *The Process of teaching the submissive to assume certain positions on command.*

Power Exchange *A defining characteristic of BDSM best described as "eroticism based on a consensual exchange of power." Empowerment of the dominant by the submissive's surrender of control to them. This relationship may be for a predetermined time, or indefinite.*

Psychodrama *Very intense form of role-playing.*

Rimming *Slang term for engaging in anal-oral sex.*

Role-Playing *The enactment of a prearranged scene wherein the two players assume characters different from their own to better play out the fantasy.*

Sadism *The act of administering pain for sensual or sexual pleasure.*

Sadist *One who gets sexual pleasure from inflicting emotional or physical pain, (extreme sensation), on others.*

Safe Word *A previously agreed upon code word to slow down or stop the scene. For example: "Red" means stop, "yellow" means slow down. "Mercy" and/or "pity" are popular.*

Sensory Deprivation *The taking away of one or more of the submissive's senses to heighten his awareness of the others.*

Sensation Play *Any BDSM activity involving creating unusual sensations on a person, who may be blindfolded, as with ice cubes, soft fur or cloth, coarse materials and the like. Sensation play is generally more mild than pain play, but can lead up to extreme sensations that can be described as erotically painful.*

Services *The many things your submissive can do for you, the dominant.*

Slave *Someone committed to the BDSM lifestyle, putting his/her entire being in her Mistress/Master's control and care. A human being who, in a fantasy, is owned as property by another and is absolutely subject to their will; a person who is completely dominated by some outside influence, habit, or another person. Note: they are more rare than purported.*

Slave Training *The process of teaching a submissive to serve a dominant.*

Soft Limits *Something that someone is hesitant or nervous about doing but would like to try if they feel they are safe with you. For these people, you need to go slowly.*

Spanking *Good old-fashioned hand-walloping delivered to the sub's bottom.*

Spreader Bar *Strong bar of wood, metal, or other material, with rings and cuffs attached to it to keep the sub's arms and/or legs apart.*

Sub Drop *A physical condition sometimes experienced by the receiver after an intense session of BDSM play, best prevented by providing aftercare immediately following the session.*

Submissive (adj.) *Having the tendency to submit without resistance; docile.*

Submissive *Someone who likes to be sexually submissive or passive. Someone who surrenders control to a dominant partner. Can also be service-oriented without any overt sexual activity. The person that surrenders control either during a scene or all the time to another during erotic play.*

Sub Space *A "natural high" or endorphin rush that a sub can get during a scene.*

Switch *These are sexual beings that can play the top or bottom, dominant or submissive, and move fluidly between the two at any given time.*

Tease and Denial *Keeping another person aroused while delaying or preventing resolution of the feelings (orgasm), to keep them in a continual state of anticipatory tension and inner conflict and heightened sensitivity.*

Top *Someone who can play the dominant role when required, usually only for certain situations, regardless of his/her orientation.*

Top Drop *Similar to "Sub Drop," but can affect a dominant or top after a scene. Feelings of guilt are commonly associated with it, and aftercare helps counteract this.*

Topping From The Bottom *The taking control of a scene by the submissive person without attempting to preserve the illusion that the dominant is in charge.*

Total Power Exchange *An energy exchange wherein the submissive gives over their power to the top or dominant in order to create an intense energy flow.*

Training *Refers to either a short or ongoing period of time in which the dominant teaches the sub how to act in a specific situation. Can either be playful or serious, depending on the couple's dynamic.*

Trigger *An emotional, mental or physical activity that causes a distinct reaction.*

Vampire Gloves *Leather gloves used for sensation play which have a large number of short spikes or needles protruding from the palms and/or fingers.*

Vanilla Sex *Term used by players for the sexual habits of non-BDSM folk and/or kinksters.*

Voyeur *One who has an interest in viewing sexual objects or activities to obtain sexual excitement whether or not the other person knows of the viewing.*

Wartenberg Wheel *A small implement consisting of a short handle to which is affixed a small wheel with a number of sharp needle-like projections around its outer edge. Used by neurologists to test nerve function in the skin and by people in the BDSM community for sensation play.*

Water Sports *Sex play involving pee.*

Weights *Lead fishing weights or other weights hung from clamps, straps, or ropes that are attached to the body for increased sensation.*

Wrapping *Curling of a whip around a part of the body not intended to be hit.*

DISCLAIMER

Although we've made every effort to ensure that the information in this book was correct at press time, Bondassage® / Jaeleen Bennis / Eve Minax does not assume and hereby disclaims any liability to any party for any loss, damage, or disruption caused by errors or omissions, whether such errors or omissions result from negligence, accident, or any other cause.

The information in this book is meant to supplement, not replace, proper training. Bondassage advises readers to take full responsibility for their safety and know their limits. Before practicing the skills described in this book, be sure that your equipment is well maintained, and do not take risks beyond your level of experience, aptitude, training and comfort level. Please ALWAYS use and respect "Safe Words."

If you think you have found a factual error, typographical error, or other inaccuracy or omission in this book, please send an email to *jaeleen@bondassage.com* to make sure this is corrected in subsequent editions.

Have fun and play safe!

ABOUT THE AUTHORS

Jaeleen Bennis is a certified massage therapist (CMT), professional Domina, and the creator and founder of Bondassage®.

As a bodyworker, she has extensive training in several healing modalities, including Swedish, Shiatsu, Deep Tissue and Sports Massage, Acupressure, Reiki, Tantra, Shamanic Journeying and Aromatherapy. She believes that BDSM is a valid path to self-discovery and healing and that submission can be a path to the divine.

Jaeleen offers training and certification in Bondassage and Elysium, coaching, mentoring, consultations and private sessions for individuals, couples, erotic bodyworkers and professional sex educators. Please contact her at *jaeleen@bondassage. com* for more information.

You can find Jaeleen on Twitter (@jaeleenbennis).

Eve Minax is a reknowned kink presenter, a lifestyle and professional Domina and Kink Coach, and acts as Lead Staff Instructor for the Cleo Dubois Academy of SM Arts in San Francisco. She has presented on kink and sexuality at numerous conferences around the country. She has assisted Barbara Carellas in teaching Urban Tantra, and is also a certified Bondassage

Practitioner. Eve holds an MA in French and English Literatures with a Gender Studies Concentration.

Follow Eve on Twitter (@eveminax).

To learn more about Bondassage or locate a Bondassage practitioner, visit the Bondassage website at bondassage.com

ACKNOWLEDGMENTS

With deepest gratitude, I wish to thank everyone who helped with the creation of this book. Eve Minax, Hillary Johnson, Jaiya, Lorna Hannah, Jo Tigerlily. Whether you cajoled, nagged, praised, read, edited, commented, participated, listened or taught me... I appreciate you more than I can say. Thank you, thank you, thank you!

—Jaeleen

It almost goes without saying that I am indebted to Jaeleen for her ongoing no-nonsense love, support and super business savvy. Cleo, Barbara and Annie for immeasurable friendship, guidance and consideration. Bobbi for a roof and a laugh. Johnny and Ham for being my rocks and my rolls. Eva for believing in my writing all these years. And finally, to all my students and teachers out there. You know who you are:) Deep gratitude and much love to you all!

—Eve

If you enjoyed this book, please consider leaving a customer review on Amazon.com to help new readers discover Bondassage. We really appreciate your support!